PROSTATE WELLNESS:

A GUIDE FOR MEN OVER 50

DR. Brandon Walker

Table of Contents

Introduction

Understanding the Importance of Prostate Health

The prostate, a small yet mighty gland nestled beneath the bladder, often remains in the shadows of health discussions. However, as men gracefully navigate the chapters beyond 50, unraveling the profound importance of prostate health becomes paramount. At its essence, the prostate stands as a sentinel of reproductive prowess, crafting seminal fluid that not only nourishes but ferries sperm, a fundamental contributor to the intricate tapestry of human fertility. This reproductive duty, often overlooked, sets the stage for a deeper understanding of the profound connection between prostate health and the foundational aspects of life.

Delving into the physiological intricacies, the prostate's location becomes pivotal in comprehending its intricate dance with urinary function. Like a guardian wrapped around the urethra, the tube responsible for the flow of urine, the prostate exerts its influence on the symphony of the urinary system. An enlarged prostate, a condition known as benign prostatic hyperplasia (BPH), can subtly encroach upon this delicate balance. The consequence? An array of symptoms, from the persistent urge to urinate to the frustration of incomplete bladder emptying. The realization that prostate health intricately entwines with everyday functions, such as the seemingly simple act of urination, prompts a reevaluation of its significance.

Yet, the prostate's role extends beyond the realms of anatomy and physiology. It confronts the specter of various disorders, each with its unique nuances and implications.

Prostatitis, an inflammation of the prostate, emerges as a silent disruptor, introducing discomfort and pain into the equation. Meanwhile, the shadow of prostate cancer looms large, a formidable adversary that demands attention and understanding. Awareness becomes a beacon, guiding men through the intricate landscape of symptoms, screening options, and treatment considerations. In these instances, the importance of acknowledging the existence of the prostate as a dynamic organ becomes not only a matter of physical health but a journey into emotional resilience.

Quality of life, an intricate tapestry woven with threads of physical and emotional well-being, emerges as a central motif in the exploration of prostate health. Chronic conditions, such as an enlarged prostate or prostate cancer, wield the potential to disrupt the harmonious rhythm of daily life. Pain, discomfort, and the psychological toll of confronting a potentially life-altering diagnosis cast shadows over the canvas. In understanding the importance of prostate health, individuals embark on a quest to preserve and enhance their overall quality of life, striving for a balance that transcends the physical realm.

Emotional well-being, often the unsung hero in health narratives, takes center stage in the prostate health saga. A diagnosis, particularly one that involves the word "cancer," can unleash a tidal wave of emotions – fear, uncertainty, and vulnerability. Acknowledging this emotional dimension is not a detour but an integral part of the prostate health journey. Support systems, both professional and personal, become the pillars that uphold individuals as they navigate the emotional landscape, fostering resilience and empowerment.

In the mosaic of preventive health measures, the understanding of prostate health emerges as the cornerstone. It becomes the compass guiding individuals toward proactive choices, lifestyle adjustments, and routine screenings. A balanced diet, regular exercise, and the avoidance of known risk factors form the arsenal against potential adversaries. Routine checkups, often viewed as mere medical rituals, transform into gateways for early detection and intervention, reinforcing the concept that knowledge and awareness are formidable allies in the pursuit of lasting health.

In essence, understanding the importance of prostate health is an odyssey into the core of masculinity, touching upon reproductive legacy, urinary grace, the delicate balance between physical and emotional well-being, and the proactive measures that carve a path toward a vibrant, fulfilling life. Beyond the anatomical intricacies, it is an acknowledgment that the prostate is not merely a gland but a guardian of vitality, a custodian of life's intricate dance, and a beacon guiding men towards a future defined by informed choices and holistic well-being.

Overview of Changes After 50

Entering the fifth decade of life marks a significant juncture, ushering in a phase of transformations that resonate through the physical, emotional, and psychological spheres. At the forefront of these changes is the subtle but undeniable shift in hormonal dynamics, where testosterone levels begin a gradual decline. This hormonal recalibration sets in motion a series of changes, from alterations in muscle mass and bone density to shifts in metabolism. The metabolism slowdown, often accompanied by a gradual increase in body fat, prompts a reconsideration of dietary habits and the need for a more active lifestyle.

Amidst these physiological adjustments, the cardiovascular system, a stalwart companion throughout earlier years, undergoes changes that demand attention. Blood vessels may become less elastic, blood pressure can exhibit subtle elevations, and cholesterol levels may show a propensity to tip the balance toward less favorable ratios. This cardiovascular evolution underscores the importance of adopting heart-healthy practices, including regular exercise, a balanced diet, and routine checkups to monitor vital indicators.

Simultaneously, the skeletal framework undergoes transformations that warrant mindful care. Bone density, a cornerstone of skeletal strength, may decrease, increasing the susceptibility to conditions like osteoporosis. Weight-bearing exercises, adequate calcium intake, and discussions with healthcare professionals about preventive measures become pivotal components in the blueprint for skeletal well-being.

The canvas of mental and emotional well-being experiences nuanced strokes, with midlife often heralding a period of introspection and reevaluation. The demands of career and family may converge with a desire for personal fulfillment, prompting individuals to contemplate life's purpose and redefine priorities. Emotional resilience becomes a linchpin, guiding individuals through the ebb and flow of life's complexities.

As the milestone of 50 is crossed, the importance of regular health screenings gains prominence. From colorectal screenings to prostate health checkups, preventive measures become linchpins in preserving overall well-being. Awareness of potential risk factors, coupled with proactive engagement with healthcare providers, becomes an indispensable facet of this phase of life.

In essence, the overview of changes after 50 is a tapestry woven with threads of transformation and self-discovery. It calls for a nuanced understanding of the body's evolving needs, a commitment to proactive health measures, and an embrace of the emotional nuances that accompany this chapter. This period, rather than a culmination, becomes a bridge to a future defined by informed choices, resilient well-being, and the richness that comes with navigating the ever-changing landscape of life beyond the half-century mark.

Chapter 1: The Prostate Unveiled

Anatomy and Function

The prostate, often regarded as a small, unassuming gland, emerges as a central figure in male reproductive anatomy, contributing not only to fertility but also influencing urinary dynamics. Nestled just below the bladder and surrounding the urethra like a guardian, its walnut-sized presence belies its significance. The primary function of the prostate lies in reproductive alchemy – the production of seminal fluid. This fluid, a complex concoction of enzymes, proteins, and nutrients, acts as a nourishing vehicle for sperm, providing them with the essential support needed for their journey toward fertilization.

The intricate dance of the prostate extends beyond reproductive duties to influence urinary function. Wrapped around the urethra, the tube responsible for the expulsion of urine from the bladder, the prostate's positioning positions it as a key player in the symphony of micturition. However, the prostate's proximity can become a source of concern, especially with the potential for conditions like benign prostatic hyperplasia (BPH). In BPH, the prostate's enlargement can impede the smooth flow of urine, leading to a constellation of symptoms, including increased frequency, urgency, and difficulty emptying the bladder.

To comprehend the anatomy of the prostate is to navigate its lobes and zones. The gland consists of three lobes – the anterior, posterior, and lateral lobes – each with distinct functions. The posterior lobe, often the site of cancerous developments, draws particular attention in medical assessments. Zones, too, distinguish themselves – the peripheral zone, where the majority of prostate cancers originate, and the transitional zone, prone to benign growth, notably in cases of BPH.

Understanding the anatomy of the prostate extends to grasping its physiological changes over the course of a man's life. Embarking on its journey from dormancy in childhood, the prostate undergoes significant growth during puberty under the influence of hormones, particularly testosterone. However, the intricacies of aging bring about a shift in hormonal dynamics, with a gradual decline in testosterone levels after the age of 30. This hormonal recalibration sets the stage for potential alterations in the prostate, contributing to the spectrum of conditions that can emerge, including prostatitis, BPH, and prostate cancer.

In essence, the anatomy and function of the prostate weave a tale of a modest gland with profound influence. Its roles in reproductive health and urinary function paint a canvas where the threads of life's complexities intersect. Navigating this terrain involves not only understanding the physical nuances of lobes and zones but also appreciating the delicate balance that ensures the prostate's harmonious coexistence within the intricate landscape of the male body.

Common Prostate Conditions Explained

The prostate, a small gland with outsized importance in male health, is susceptible to a spectrum of conditions that can significantly impact well-being. Understanding these common prostate conditions is pivotal for men navigating the terrain of urological health beyond the age of 50.

1. **Benign Prostatic Hyperplasia (BPH):**

   Benign Prostatic Hyperplasia (BPH), a common and non-cancerous condition affecting the prostate, stands as a testament to the intricate dance between aging and male reproductive health. As men venture into their later years, the prostate, a gland initially modest in size, undergoes a transformation, gradually enlarging and introducing the complexities of BPH.

   The genesis of BPH lies in the subtle hormonal shifts that accompany the aging process. Testosterone, the primary male sex hormone, experiences a gradual decline after the age of 30. While this decrease is a natural facet of aging, it can trigger the proliferation of prostate cells, leading to the enlargement of the gland. This expansion primarily occurs in the transitional zone of the prostate, the area surrounding the urethra, which becomes the focal point for BPH-related symptoms.

   The symptoms of BPH can manifest gradually, often masquerading as typical signs of aging. Increased urinary frequency, especially during the night (nocturia), a sense of urgency to urinate, and a weakened urine stream are common indicators of an enlarging prostate. As the prostate encroaches on the urethra, it creates a scenario where the bladder must exert more force to expel urine, leading to these characteristic symptoms.

Navigating the landscape of BPH involves not only recognizing the symptoms but also understanding the potential impact on daily life. The condition can introduce challenges such as frequent interruptions to sleep due to nocturia, an increased risk of urinary tract infections, and a diminished quality of life if left unaddressed. Furthermore, BPH can create a cycle of anxiety and frustration as individuals grapple with the disruptive influence it has on their urinary habits.

Diagnosing BPH typically involves a comprehensive assessment, beginning with a detailed medical history and physical examination. The International Prostate Symptom Score (IPSS) questionnaire may be utilized to gauge the severity of symptoms, and additional tests, such as a prostate-specific antigen (PSA) blood test and a digital rectal exam, may be conducted to rule out other potential issues, including prostate cancer.

Treatment strategies for BPH span a spectrum, ranging from lifestyle modifications to medical interventions. Lifestyle adjustments often include dietary changes, such as reducing caffeine and alcohol intake, managing fluid consumption, and engaging in regular physical activity. Medications, such as alpha-blockers or 5-alpha reductase inhibitors, may be prescribed to alleviate symptoms by relaxing the muscles around the prostate or reducing its size.

For cases resistant to conservative measures, surgical interventions may be considered. Transurethral Resection of the Prostate (TURP), GreenLight Laser Therapy, and other minimally invasive procedures aim to relieve symptoms by removing excess prostate tissue.

The journey through BPH, though common, is unique for each individual. It demands a nuanced approach that considers not only the physical manifestations of the condition but also its impact on the emotional and psychological well-being of those affected. Open communication with healthcare providers, regular checkups, and a proactive stance toward one's health become instrumental in navigating the landscape of an enlarged prostate. BPH, while presenting challenges, underscores the resilience of individuals in adapting to the changes that accompany the aging process, forging a path toward a life characterized by informed choices and sustained well-being.

2. **Prostatitis: Decoding the Intricacies of Inflammation in the Prostate**

As a urologist, addressing prostatitis requires a comprehensive understanding of the nuances surrounding this intricate and often challenging condition. Prostatitis, characterized by inflammation of the prostate gland, presents a spectrum of clinical scenarios, each necessitating a tailored approach to diagnosis and management.

Classification and Presentation:

Prostatitis is classified into several subtypes, including acute bacterial prostatitis, chronic bacterial prostatitis, chronic pelvic pain syndrome (CPPS), and asymptomatic inflammatory prostatitis. Each subtype exhibits distinct clinical features and poses unique challenges. Acute bacterial prostatitis manifests with sudden-onset severe symptoms, including fever, chills, and perineal or pelvic pain. Chronic bacterial prostatitis is marked by recurrent urinary tract infections. Chronic pelvic pain syndrome is the most common, presenting with persistent pelvic pain, discomfort, and urinary symptoms, often lacking a clear bacterial etiology.

Diagnostic Challenges:

Diagnosing prostatitis requires a judicious blend of medical history, clinical examination, and laboratory investigations. Differentiating between the subtypes is crucial for tailored management. The National Institutes of Health Chronic Prostatitis Symptom Index (NIH-CPSI) serves as a valuable tool in assessing the severity and impact of symptoms in chronic cases. Laboratory studies, including urine cultures and prostate-specific antigen (PSA) tests, aid in ruling out bacterial involvement and prostate cancer.

Management Strategies:

The treatment approach to prostatitis hinges on the specific subtype identified. Acute bacterial prostatitis typically necessitates prompt initiation of broad-spectrum antibiotics, followed by targeted therapy based on culture results. Chronic bacterial prostatitis requires prolonged courses of antibiotics to eradicate persistent infections. In chronic pelvic pain syndrome, a multidisciplinary approach is often employed. Alpha-blockers, anti-inflammatory medications, and pelvic floor physical therapy may be integral components of management.

Challenges in Chronic Pelvic Pain Syndrome (CPPS):

Chronic pelvic pain syndrome poses unique challenges due to its complex etiology, which may involve inflammatory, neuromuscular, and psychological factors. Management often requires a patient-centered approach, involving education, lifestyle modifications, and pharmacotherapy. Addressing psychological factors, such as stress and anxiety, is crucial in achieving comprehensive symptom relief.

Prognosis and Follow-up:

Prostatitis can have varying prognoses depending on the subtype and the effectiveness of the chosen intervention. Acute bacterial prostatitis, when promptly treated, typically resolves with a favorable prognosis. Chronic cases, especially those involving pelvic pain syndrome, may necessitate long-term management and periodic follow-ups to assess response to treatment and adjust therapeutic strategies accordingly.

Navigating prostatitis as a urologist involves not only deciphering its clinical intricacies but also fostering a patient-centric approach that acknowledges the impact of symptoms on an individual's quality of life. In the realm of prostatitis, the urologist serves as a guide, steering patients through the complexities of diagnosis, offering tailored therapeutic interventions, and cultivating an ongoing partnership in the journey towards sustained urological health. Prostatitis, though challenging, provides an opportunity for urologists to showcase the depth of their expertise and compassion, underscoring the commitment to enhancing the well-being of those entrusted to their care.

Case Study: Unraveling the Complexities of Prostatitis in Patient X

Patient X, a 42-year-old male, presented to the urology clinic with a chief complaint of persistent pelvic pain, discomfort during urination, and a sense of urgency. The nuanced case unveiled a scenario that would later be diagnosed as chronic pelvic pain syndrome (CPPS), a subtype of prostatitis that often challenges both patients and urologists due to its multifactorial nature.

1. **Symptomatology and Initial Assessment:** Patient X's journey began with symptoms of discomfort and occasional pelvic pain that had gradually intensified over the preceding six months. A detailed medical history highlighted the absence of urinary tract infections or other identifiable causes, suggesting a non-bacterial etiology. The National Institutes of Health Chronic Prostatitis Symptom Index (NIH-CPSI) revealed a moderate to severe impact on the patient's quality of life, particularly in terms of pain severity and urinary symptoms.

2. **Diagnostic Challenges:** Despite the absence of clear bacterial markers, a thorough diagnostic workup was initiated. Urine cultures ruled out bacterial prostatitis, and a prostate-specific antigen (PSA) test returned within normal limits. Imaging studies, including transrectal ultrasound, provided insights into prostate size and structure. The diagnosis of chronic pelvic pain syndrome (CPPS) was solidified based on the clinical presentation, negative bacterial studies, and the characteristic findings on imaging.

3. **Multidisciplinary Approach to Management:** Patient X's case underscored the need for a multidisciplinary approach. Collaborating with colleagues in pain management and psychology, the urologist implemented a tailored treatment plan. Alpha-blockers were initiated to alleviate urinary symptoms, while anti-inflammatory medications provided relief for pelvic pain. Concurrently, pelvic

floor physical therapy was incorporated to address potential neuromuscular factors contributing to the symptoms.

4. **Psychological Support and Coping Strategies:** Recognizing the intertwined nature of psychological factors in CPPS, Patient X was offered psychological support to address stress and anxiety associated with chronic pain. Education played a pivotal role in empowering the patient to understand the chronic nature of CPPS and adopting coping strategies to enhance resilience.

5. **Ongoing Follow-up and Adjustments:** Patient X's response to the initial treatment was encouraging, with a notable reduction in pain and improvement in urinary symptoms. However, the chronic nature of CPPS necessitated ongoing follow-up to monitor symptom fluctuations and make adjustments to the treatment plan as needed. Patient education remained a cornerstone, enabling Patient X to actively participate in managing his condition.

This case study illustrates the intricacies inherent in diagnosing and managing chronic pelvic pain syndrome, a subtype of prostatitis. It emphasizes the importance of a thorough diagnostic evaluation, a multidisciplinary treatment approach, and ongoing collaboration between the patient and healthcare team. Patient X's journey reflects the challenges posed by prostatitis and highlights the nuanced role of urologists in navigating these complexities to achieve comprehensive and patient-centered care.

3. **Prostate Cancer:**

Prostate cancer, a formidable adversary in the realm of men's health, demands a meticulous understanding of its complexities and a nuanced approach to diagnosis and management. As a urologist, encountering patients like Mr. Y, a 60-year-old individual with an elevated prostate-specific antigen (PSA) level and concerning findings on digital rectal examination, underscores the gravity of this silent threat. Prostate cancer often presents insidiously, with subtle or absent symptoms in its early stages, making routine screening imperative, especially for those in their sixth decade and beyond.

In Mr. Y's case, the initial diagnostic journey involved a comprehensive evaluation. The PSA test, while a valuable screening tool, prompted further investigation. Prostate biopsies were performed to assess tissue samples, allowing for the identification of cancerous cells and determination of the cancer's aggressiveness through grading systems like the Gleason score. Imaging studies, such as multiparametric magnetic resonance imaging (mpMRI), played a crucial role in staging the cancer, guiding treatment decisions, and estimating the extent of disease spread.

The management of prostate cancer encompasses a spectrum of options, each tailored to the unique characteristics of the individual case. For localized or low-grade tumors, active surveillance may be a viable approach, involving close monitoring with periodic PSA tests and biopsies. Conversely, more aggressive cases may necessitate definitive interventions such as surgery (radical prostatectomy) or radiation therapy. For advanced prostate cancer, systemic treatments like hormone therapy, chemotherapy, or novel targeted therapies may be employed to manage the disease and alleviate symptoms.

Navigating the landscape of prostate cancer involves not only addressing the physical aspects of the disease but also acknowledging its profound impact on the emotional and psychological well-being of patients. Mr. Y's case exemplifies the importance of open communication, patient education, and a shared decision-making process. Discussing the potential side effects of treatment, addressing concerns about quality of life, and involving the patient in the decision-making process are integral components of the holistic care paradigm.

The role of a urologist extends beyond diagnosis and treatment to survivorship care and ongoing monitoring. Post-treatment follow-ups, involving regular PSA tests and clinical assessments, are crucial for detecting potential recurrences or treatment-related complications. Additionally, the urologist collaborates with other healthcare professionals, including oncologists and radiologists, to ensure a comprehensive and coordinated approach to prostate cancer care.

In essence, prostate cancer demands a vigilant and multidisciplinary stance. For urologists, it represents a dynamic landscape where early detection, personalized treatment strategies, and ongoing support converge to offer the best possible outcomes. The case of Mr. Y exemplifies the intricate nature of prostate cancer care, emphasizing the importance of tailored approaches, informed decision-making, and a holistic perspective that extends beyond the physical manifestations of the disease.

4. Prostatic Intraepithelial Neoplasia (PIN):

Prostatic Intraepithelial Neoplasia (PIN) serves as a critical waypoint in the landscape of prostate health, offering a glimpse into potential precursors to prostate cancer. As a urologist, encounters with patients like Mr. Z, a 55-year-old male with elevated PSA levels and an incidental finding of high-grade PIN on prostate biopsy, highlight the significance of understanding and addressing these early cellular changes. PIN is characterized by the presence of abnormal cells within the prostate ducts, and while it is not cancer itself, high-grade PIN is recognized as a potential precursor to invasive prostate cancer.

The diagnostic journey in cases of high-grade PIN often begins with an elevation in PSA levels, prompting further investigation to identify potential underlying causes. In Mr. Z's case, a prostate biopsy revealed the presence of high-grade PIN, raising concerns about the risk of progression to prostate cancer. The focus then shifts to risk stratification and determining the appropriate course of action. Additional diagnostic tools, including imaging studies and repeated biopsies, may be employed to gather more information about the extent of PIN and assess the overall health of the prostate.

Managing high-grade PIN requires a nuanced approach, balancing the need for vigilance with the understanding that not all cases progress to cancer. For patients like Mr. Z, close monitoring becomes a cornerstone of care. Regular follow-ups, involving PSA tests and periodic biopsies, allow urologists to track changes over time and identify any signs of progression. Patient education is pivotal, as individuals need to comprehend the nature of high-grade PIN, its potential implications, and the rationale behind the chosen management strategy.

The urologist's role extends beyond diagnosis and monitoring to actively engaging with patients in shared decision-making. For individuals with high-grade PIN, considerations for lifestyle modifications, such as adopting a heart-healthy diet and regular exercise, are often discussed. These lifestyle changes, while not guaranteed to prevent cancer, are associated with overall health benefits and may contribute to prostate health. The urologist serves as a guide, offering support and information to empower patients in making informed choices about their health.

Understanding the natural history of high-grade PIN involves acknowledging its variability and the inherent uncertainty surrounding its progression. Some cases may remain stable or regress over time, while others may evolve into prostate cancer. This complexity necessitates ongoing communication between the urologist and the patient, fostering a relationship built on trust and collaboration. In Mr. Z's case, the urologist plays a pivotal role in providing reassurance, answering questions, and addressing any concerns that may arise during the monitoring process.

The landscape of high-grade PIN underscores the evolving nature of prostate health and the importance of precision medicine in urology. Advances in molecular and genetic profiling may offer insights into the likelihood of progression and guide personalized management strategies. Urologists, as stewards of prostate health, stay at the forefront of these developments, integrating them into the overall care paradigm for patients with high-grade PIN.

In conclusion, high-grade PIN represents a critical juncture in the journey of prostate health. For urologists, it embodies the delicate balance between vigilance and restraint, offering an opportunity to intervene early while acknowledging the inherent uncertainties. The case of Mr. Z exemplifies the urologist's role as a collaborator, educator, and advocate, navigating the landscape of high-grade PIN with precision and compassion.

5. **Chronic Prostatitis/Chronic Pelvic Pain Syndrome (CP/CPPS):**

Chronic Prostatitis/Chronic Pelvic Pain Syndrome (CP/CPPS) emerges as a perplexing entity within the realm of urological health, challenging both patients and urologists due to its chronicity and multifactorial nature. Consider the case of Mr. A, a 48-year-old male who presented with recurrent pelvic pain, discomfort during urination, and an overall diminished quality of life. This subtype of prostatitis, characterized by persistent pelvic pain lasting for at least three months, often lacks a clear bacterial cause, adding layers of complexity to its diagnosis and management.

Symptomatology and Diagnostic Exploration:

Mr. A's journey began with the manifestation of pelvic pain, discomfort, and urinary symptoms that persisted over several months. The absence of clear evidence of bacterial infection prompted the consideration of CP/CPPS. The National Institutes of Health Chronic Prostatitis Symptom Index (NIH-CPSI) became a valuable tool in quantifying the severity and impact of Mr. A's symptoms. Other diagnostic measures, including urine cultures, ruled out bacterial involvement, reinforcing the diagnosis of a chronic nonbacterial prostatitis.

Multifaceted Etiology and Contributing Factors:

CP/CPPS poses a diagnostic challenge due to its multifactorial etiology. While bacterial infections are excluded, various contributing factors come into play, including neuromuscular dysfunction, psychological stressors, and immunological responses. Understanding the interplay of these factors becomes essential in crafting a comprehensive management plan for patients like Mr. A.

Multidisciplinary Approach to Management:

The management of CP/CPPS demands a multidisciplinary approach that goes beyond traditional urological interventions. Mr. A's treatment plan involved a combination of pharmacotherapy, including alpha-blockers and anti-inflammatory medications, to alleviate symptoms.

Additionally, pelvic floor physical therapy was integrated to address potential neuromuscular components contributing to his discomfort. Psychological support, acknowledging the emotional toll of chronic pain, became an integral part of Mr. A's care.

Patient Education and Coping Strategies:

Educating patients about the chronic nature of CP/CPPS and involving them in the decision-making process are crucial aspects of care. Mr. A's urologist played a pivotal role in providing information about the condition, discussing potential triggers, and empowering him with coping strategies. Lifestyle modifications, stress management techniques, and relaxation exercises were introduced to enhance Mr. A's ability to navigate the challenges of living with chronic pelvic pain.

Long-Term Follow-up and Adaptations:

CP/CPPS often requires ongoing follow-up and adaptability in the management plan. Regular assessments, including NIH-CPSI scores and discussions about symptom fluctuations, are essential for refining the approach over time. For patients like Mr. A, the urologist becomes a partner in the long-term journey, adjusting interventions based on the patient's response and evolving needs.

In essence, chronic prostatitis/chronic pelvic pain syndrome unfolds as a complex puzzle within urological practice. The case of Mr. A exemplifies the intricate nature of CP/CPPS, highlighting the need for a patient-centered approach, ongoing collaboration between the healthcare team and the patient, and a holistic perspective that extends beyond the traditional boundaries of urological care. The urologist, in navigating the enigma of CP/CPPS, emerges as a guide, advocate, and partner in the quest for sustained well-being for individuals living with chronic pelvic discomfort.

Understanding these common prostate conditions involves recognizing their distinct characteristics, symptoms, and potential impact on daily life. While BPH and prostatitis may cause bothersome urinary symptoms, prostate cancer introduces the specter of a potentially life-threatening disease. Timely medical attention, regular checkups, and open communication with healthcare providers are crucial components in the proactive management of these conditions. Additionally, the nuances of each condition necessitate tailored approaches to diagnosis and treatment, underlining the importance of personalized care in addressing prostate health concerns.

Chapter 2: Age-Related Changes

Hormonal Shifts and Their Impact

Hormonal shifts in men, particularly the gradual decline in testosterone levels as they age, intricately weave into the fabric of their overall health, ushering in a phase marked by both subtle and pronounced transformations. This hormonal ebb and flow, often beginning around the age of 30, orchestrates a symphony of physiological changes that reverberate through various facets of well-being.

Muscle mass, a cornerstone of physical strength, faces the inevitable consequences of hormonal fluctuations. As testosterone levels decline, the body's ability to maintain and build muscle diminishes, leading to a gradual reduction in muscle mass. This not only alters body composition but also contributes to the challenges of weight management and metabolic health. The interplay between hormonal shifts and metabolism becomes particularly pronounced, with a potential slowing down of metabolic processes that can lead to changes in weight distribution and an increased risk of metabolic conditions such as insulin resistance.

Simultaneously, bone density undergoes transformations, presenting a significant concern for skeletal health. Testosterone plays a crucial role in maintaining bone density, and its decline can contribute to decreased bone mass, ultimately elevating the risk of osteoporosis. The skeletal framework, a structural foundation for overall well-being, becomes susceptible to fractures and fractures, emphasizing the importance of proactive measures such as weight-bearing exercises and adequate calcium intake to fortify bone health.

In the realm of reproductive health, hormonal shifts set the stage for potential challenges. The prostate gland, situated at the crossroads of hormonal regulation, responds to these changes with implications for men's health. The delicate balance between the benefits of testosterone and the potential risks emerges, with conditions such as benign prostatic hyperplasia (BPH) and prostate cancer gaining prominence. While BPH results from the non-cancerous enlargement of the prostate, prostate cancer poses a more formidable threat, often linked to age-related hormonal changes. The impact of hormonal shifts on prostate health underscores the importance of regular screenings and proactive engagement with healthcare providers to detect and manage potential concerns.

Beyond the physical realm, hormonal fluctuations cast their influence on mental and emotional well-being. Mood swings, fatigue, and changes in cognitive function can be attributed, in part, to hormonal changes. The intricate interplay between hormones and neurotransmitters shapes the emotional landscape, prompting individuals to navigate through the nuanced complexities of mental health. Recognizing these emotional nuances becomes pivotal, fostering an environment where emotional well-being is acknowledged and addressed alongside physical health.

Understanding the profound repercussions of hormonal shifts is a cornerstone of holistic healthcare for men as they age. Proactive measures become instrumental in mitigating potential risks and enhancing overall well-being. Regular exercise, tailored nutritional strategies, and stress management techniques stand as pillars in navigating the dynamic terrain of hormonal fluctuations. Lifestyle modifications, when implemented early and consistently, can contribute to maintaining muscle mass, supporting bone health, and fostering emotional resilience.

As men traverse the journey of aging, a comprehensive approach to healthcare becomes paramount. Regular health checkups, including assessments of hormonal levels, provide a roadmap for personalized interventions. Collaborative efforts between individuals and healthcare providers facilitate informed decision-making, ensuring that the impact of hormonal shifts is managed effectively. Embracing the dynamic nature of hormonal changes, rather than viewing them as inevitable adversaries, allows for a proactive and empowered approach to aging gracefully and maintaining optimal well-being throughout the different seasons of life.

Recognizing Normal vs. Concerning Symptoms

Recognizing normal versus concerning symptoms is a critical aspect of self-awareness and proactive healthcare, enabling individuals to distinguish between the expected fluctuations in well-being and potential indicators of underlying health issues. Normal symptoms often align with the body's natural responses to various factors, including lifestyle, aging, and environmental influences. For instance, occasional fluctuations in energy levels, mood, or sleep patterns are part of the normal spectrum, influenced by factors such as stress, daily activities, and sleep hygiene. Similarly, subtle changes in weight, appetite, or bowel habits may reflect the body's adaptive responses to dietary variations and lifestyle choices. Understanding and acknowledging these variations contribute to a comprehensive understanding of one's baseline health.

On the other hand, concerning symptoms demand closer attention and prompt medical evaluation. Persistent or severe deviations from one's normal state may signify underlying health conditions that require intervention. For example, unexplained weight loss, especially when coupled with changes in appetite, can be indicative of various health issues, including metabolic disorders or gastrointestinal conditions. Unrelenting fatigue, beyond what is expected from daily activities or inadequate sleep, may raise concerns about systemic conditions such as anemia, thyroid disorders, or chronic fatigue syndrome. Recognizing the distinction between normal fluctuations and concerning symptoms is crucial in fostering a proactive approach to health.

In the realm of cardiovascular health, understanding the difference between normal aging-related changes and potential warning signs is pivotal. Gradual decreases in cardiovascular fitness, endurance, and muscle mass are expected as individuals age. However, recognizing concerning symptoms such as persistent chest pain, shortness of breath, or irregular heartbeats is paramount. These symptoms could indicate cardiovascular issues, including heart disease or arrhythmias, necessitating immediate medical attention. Regular cardiovascular screenings, awareness of risk factors, and prompt reporting of unusual symptoms empower individuals to distinguish between the expected effects of aging on the cardiovascular system and potential indicators of cardiovascular diseases.

In the context of mental health, recognizing the spectrum of normal emotions and stress responses is crucial. Feeling occasional stress, sadness, or anxiety is a normal part of the human experience, influenced by life events and daily challenges. However, persistent, intense, or unmanageable symptoms may signal mental health concerns such as depression or anxiety disorders. Changes in sleep patterns, appetite, or social behaviors that disrupt daily functioning should be considered as potential red flags. Recognizing the line between normal emotional variations and concerning symptoms enables individuals to seek timely mental health support, fostering resilience and overall well-being.

In the realm of gastrointestinal health, understanding the nuances of digestive patterns aids in distinguishing between normal variations and potential gastrointestinal disorders. Occasional changes in bowel habits, influenced by diet and lifestyle, are expected. However, persistent alterations such as prolonged diarrhea, constipation, or blood in the stool merit attention. These symptoms could be indicative of conditions such as inflammatory bowel disease, irritable bowel syndrome, or colorectal cancer. Recognizing the significance of concerning gastrointestinal symptoms allows individuals to engage in proactive health-seeking behaviors, such as screenings and consultations with healthcare providers.

In the context of reproductive health, recognizing normal variations and concerning symptoms is crucial for both men and women. For women, understanding the menstrual cycle and its fluctuations helps distinguish between normal hormonal changes and potential reproductive health issues. Irregularities in menstrual patterns, persistent pelvic pain, or abnormal bleeding may signal conditions such as polycystic ovary syndrome (PCOS) or endometriosis. For men, changes in sexual function, such as erectile dysfunction or alterations in libido, could be indicative of underlying conditions like hormonal imbalances or cardiovascular issues. Acknowledging these variations encourages open communication with healthcare providers, facilitating early detection and intervention when necessary.

Overall, the ability to recognize normal versus concerning symptoms forms the foundation of proactive healthcare.

Regular health assessments, self-monitoring, and an informed awareness of one's body contribute to a holistic approach to well-being. Cultivating a health-conscious mindset involves understanding the expected variations in different aspects of health, coupled with a keen awareness of symptoms that may signal potential health issues. This proactive stance empowers individuals to engage in timely medical consultations, screenings, and lifestyle modifications, fostering a resilient and informed approach to maintaining optimal health across the lifespan.

Chapter 3: Lifestyle and Nutrition

Prostate-Friendly Diet and Nutrition Tips

Adopting a prostate-friendly diet is an essential aspect of promoting prostate health and reducing the risk of prostate-related issues, including benign prostatic hyperplasia (BPH) and prostate cancer. Here are some nutrition tips to support prostate health:

1. **Focus on Fruits and Vegetables:** Incorporate a variety of fruits and vegetables into your daily meals. These foods are rich in antioxidants, vitamins, and minerals that contribute to overall health. Cruciferous vegetables like broccoli, cauliflower, and Brussels sprouts, in particular, contain compounds that may have protective effects on the prostate.

2. **Include Tomatoes and Berries:** Tomatoes are a valuable source of lycopene, a potent antioxidant associated with prostate health. Cooked or processed tomatoes, as in tomato sauce or puree, contain higher levels of lycopene. Berries, such as strawberries, blueberries, and raspberries, provide additional antioxidants that can support overall well-being.

3. **Incorporate Healthy Fats:** Opt for sources of healthy fats, such as those found in fatty fish (salmon, trout, and sardines), flaxseeds, chia seeds, and walnuts. Omega-3 fatty acids, in particular, have anti-inflammatory properties that may contribute to prostate health.

4. **Choose Lean Protein:** Include lean protein sources in your diet, such as poultry, fish, tofu, and legumes. Limit red meat consumption, especially processed meats, as high intake has been associated with an increased risk of prostate cancer.

5. **Embrace Whole Grains:** Choose whole grains over refined carbohydrates. Whole grains like brown rice, quinoa, and whole wheat provide fiber, vitamins, and minerals that contribute to overall health and may have protective effects on the prostate.

6. **Moderate Dairy Intake:** If you consume dairy, opt for low-fat or fat-free options. Some studies suggest a potential link between high intake of dairy, especially whole milk, and an increased risk of prostate cancer. However, more research is needed in this area.

7. **Stay Hydrated:** Adequate hydration is crucial for overall health. Water helps in flushing out toxins from the body and supports proper bodily functions. Limiting caffeine and alcohol intake can also contribute to better prostate health.

8. **Watch Your Calcium Levels:** While calcium is essential for bone health, excessive intake, especially from supplements, may be associated with an increased risk of prostate cancer. Aim to meet your calcium needs through dietary sources rather than supplements.

9. **Maintain a Healthy Weight:** Obesity has been linked to an increased risk of prostate-related issues. Adopting a balanced diet and staying physically

active can help maintain a healthy weight and reduce the risk of prostate problems.

10. **Limit Added Sugars and Processed Foods:** High intake of added sugars and processed foods may contribute to inflammation and other health issues. Focus on whole, nutrient-dense foods to provide essential vitamins and minerals without unnecessary additives.

It's essential to note that individual dietary needs may vary, and consulting with a healthcare provider or a registered dietitian can provide personalized guidance based on specific health conditions and goals. Additionally, a prostate-friendly diet is just one aspect of maintaining overall health, and adopting a healthy lifestyle that includes regular physical activity, stress management, and regular medical check-ups is crucial for comprehensive well-being.

ONE WEEK PROSTATE FRIENDLY RECIPE

Here's a one-week meal plan with recipes that incorporate foods believed to support prostate health. Remember to consult with a healthcare professional or a registered dietitian for personalized advice based on your individual health needs.

Day 1:

Breakfast: Smoothie with:

- 1 cup mixed berries (blueberries, strawberries, raspberries)

- 1 banana

- 1 tablespoon flaxseeds

- 1/2 cup Greek yogurt

- 1 cup almond milk

Lunch: Grilled Salmon Salad:

- Grilled salmon fillet

- Mixed greens (spinach, kale, arugula)

- Cherry tomatoes

- Cucumber slices

- Avocado

- Olive oil and lemon dressing

Dinner: Quinoa-Stuffed Bell Peppers:

- Bell peppers stuffed with a mix of cooked quinoa, black beans, diced tomatoes, and spices

- Baked until peppers are tender

- Served with a side of steamed broccoli

Day 2:

Breakfast: Oatmeal with Walnuts and Berries:

- 1 cup cooked oats

- Handful of walnuts

- Fresh berries (blueberries or raspberries)

- Drizzle of honey

Lunch: Turkey and Avocado Wrap:

- Whole-grain wrap filled with lean turkey slices, avocado, lettuce, and tomato

- Served with a side of carrot sticks

Dinner: Baked Chicken Breast with Sweet Potato:

- Seasoned chicken breast baked until golden

- Roasted sweet potato wedges

- Steamed green beans

Day 3:

Breakfast: Greek Yogurt Parfait:

- Layered Greek yogurt with granola, sliced almonds, and fresh mango

Lunch: Quinoa Salad with Chickpeas:

- Quinoa salad with chickpeas, cherry tomatoes, cucumber, feta cheese, and a lemon-tahini dressing

Dinner: Vegetarian Stir-Fry:

- Tofu or tempeh stir-fried with broccoli, bell peppers, snap peas, and carrots

- Served over brown rice

Day 4:

Breakfast: Whole Grain Toast with Avocado:

- Whole grain toast topped with mashed avocado, cherry tomatoes, and a sprinkle of pumpkin seeds

Lunch: Mediterranean Salad with Grilled Chicken:

- Mixed greens with grilled chicken, cherry tomatoes, olives, feta cheese, and balsamic vinaigrette

Dinner: Salmon with Asparagus and Quinoa:

- Baked salmon fillet with a side of roasted asparagus and quinoa

Day 5:

Breakfast: Smoothie Bowl:

- Blended frozen berries, banana, spinach, and almond milk

- Topped with granola, sliced almonds, and chia seeds

Lunch: Chickpea and Vegetable Wrap:

- Whole-grain wrap filled with chickpeas, hummus, spinach, cucumber, and tomato

Dinner: Grilled Shrimp Skewers with Brown Rice:

- Marinated shrimp grilled on skewers

- Served with a side of brown rice and steamed broccoli

Day 6:

Breakfast: Chia Seed Pudding:

- Chia seeds soaked in almond milk overnight

- Topped with sliced kiwi, strawberries, and a drizzle of honey

Lunch: Turkey and Quinoa Stuffed Peppers:

- Bell peppers stuffed with a mix of cooked quinoa, lean ground turkey, black beans, and spices

- Baked until peppers are tender

Dinner: Vegetable and Lentil Soup:

- Hearty soup with lentils, carrots, celery, tomatoes, and kale

- Served with a side of whole-grain bread

Day 7:

Breakfast: Whole Grain Pancakes with Berries:

- Whole grain pancakes topped with fresh berries and a dollop of Greek yogurt

Lunch: Spinach and Feta Omelette:

- Omelette filled with spinach, feta cheese, and cherry tomatoes

- Served with a side of whole-grain toast

Dinner: Grilled Veggie and Chicken Skewers:

- Skewers with grilled chicken, zucchini, cherry tomatoes, and mushrooms

- Quinoa on the side

Remember to drink plenty of water throughout the day and adjust portion sizes based on individual needs. This meal plan incorporates a variety of nutrient-dense foods that are believed to be beneficial for prostate health. However, it's crucial to maintain a balanced diet, engage in regular physical activity, and consult with healthcare professionals for personalized guidance.

The Role of Exercise in Prostate Health

Exercise plays a pivotal role in promoting prostate health and may contribute to reducing the risk of prostate-related issues such as benign prostatic hyperplasia (BPH) and prostate cancer. The impact of regular physical activity on prostate health is multifaceted, encompassing various physiological, hormonal, and immune system mechanisms. Engaging in consistent exercise is associated with maintaining a healthy body weight, and obesity is a known risk factor for prostate issues. Regular physical activity helps regulate hormones, including insulin and testosterone, creating a hormonal environment that supports overall health. Furthermore, exercise is linked to enhancing immune function, which plays a crucial role in detecting and eliminating potentially harmful cells, including those in the prostate.

Aerobic exercises, such as walking, jogging, cycling, and swimming, have been specifically associated with prostate health benefits. These activities contribute to improved cardiovascular fitness, which, in turn, supports overall blood circulation, including to the prostate gland. Enhanced blood flow facilitates the delivery of essential nutrients and oxygen to the prostate, promoting its optimal function and potentially reducing the risk of cellular abnormalities.

Resistance training, involving activities like weightlifting, is another vital component of a comprehensive exercise regimen for prostate health. Building and maintaining muscle mass through resistance training not only supports overall physical well-being but also contributes to weight management, a factor linked to reduced risks of prostate issues. Additionally, resistance training can positively influence insulin sensitivity and hormonal balance, both of which are intricately connected to prostate health.

The benefits of exercise extend beyond the physical realm, impacting psychological and emotional well-being. Regular physical activity has been shown to reduce stress and anxiety levels, which can indirectly contribute to prostate health. Stress management is crucial, as chronic stress may exacerbate inflammation in the body, potentially influencing the development and progression of prostate-related conditions.

Studies have suggested a potential link between sedentary behavior and an increased risk of prostate issues. Prolonged periods of sitting or a sedentary lifestyle may negatively impact metabolic health, hormonal balance, and overall physical fitness, creating an environment conducive to prostate problems. Incorporating breaks in sedentary activities with short bouts of physical activity, such as standing, stretching, or walking, can be beneficial for prostate health.

Prostate-specific exercises, often referred to as Kegel exercises, are designed to target the pelvic floor muscles, including those around the prostate. These exercises involve contracting and relaxing the pelvic muscles, contributing to better urinary control and potential improvements in prostate symptoms, especially for individuals with conditions like BPH. While not a substitute for a comprehensive exercise routine, prostate-specific exercises can complement overall physical activity for targeted benefits.

It's essential to note that individual exercise needs may vary, and consultation with healthcare professionals is crucial before starting a new exercise regimen, especially for individuals with existing health conditions. Tailoring exercise programs to individual fitness levels, preferences, and health status ensures a safe and effective approach to improving prostate health.

In conclusion, exercise emerges as a powerful tool in promoting prostate health through its diverse physiological and psychological benefits. Engaging in a combination of aerobic exercises, resistance training, stress management, and targeted prostate-specific exercises contributes to a holistic approach that may reduce the risk of prostate-related issues. Making regular physical activity a cornerstone of a healthy lifestyle not only fosters overall well-being but also empowers individuals to take an active role in maintaining optimal prostate health throughout different stages of life.

Chapter 4: Mind-Body Connection

Stress Management for Prostate Well-Being

Stress management plays a vital role in supporting prostate well-being, as chronic stress has been linked to various health issues, including prostate-related conditions like benign prostatic hyperplasia (BPH) and prostate cancer. Understanding the intricate relationship between stress and prostate health underscores the importance of adopting effective stress management strategies as part of a holistic approach to overall well-being.

Chronic stress can trigger physiological responses that may negatively impact the prostate. The release of stress hormones, such as cortisol, in response to prolonged stress can contribute to inflammation and immune system dysregulation, creating an environment that may influence the development and progression of prostate issues. Moreover, stress-induced behaviors, such as poor dietary choices, sedentary lifestyles, and inadequate sleep, can further compound the risk factors associated with prostate health.

Implementing stress management techniques can mitigate the potential negative effects of stress on the prostate. Mindfulness practices, including meditation and deep breathing exercises, have shown promise in reducing stress levels. These techniques promote relaxation, decrease the production of stress hormones, and enhance overall emotional well-being. Incorporating mindfulness into daily routines, even for a few minutes, can contribute to a calmer state of mind.

Regular physical activity is another effective stress management tool with direct benefits for prostate health. Exercise stimulates the release of endorphins, the body's natural mood enhancers, promoting a sense of well-being and reducing stress levels. Engaging in activities such as walking, jogging, or yoga not only contributes to physical fitness but also serves as a valuable outlet for stress reduction.

Social connections and support networks are crucial components of stress management. Building and maintaining positive relationships with friends, family, or support groups provide avenues for expressing emotions, sharing concerns, and receiving encouragement. The sense of connection and understanding derived from social interactions can alleviate feelings of isolation and contribute to a more resilient response to stress.

Adequate sleep is often underestimated in its role as a stress management tool and a factor in prostate health. Sleep is a critical time for the body to repair and regenerate, and disruptions in sleep patterns can exacerbate stress levels. Establishing a consistent sleep routine, creating a comfortable sleep environment, and practicing relaxation techniques before bedtime can contribute to better sleep quality.

Cognitive-behavioral strategies, including stress-reducing techniques and positive affirmations, can help individuals reframe their perceptions of stressors. Developing resilience in the face of life's challenges can empower individuals to navigate stress more effectively, minimizing its potential impact on both mental and physical health.

Nutrition also plays a role in stress management and prostate health. Adopting a well-balanced diet that includes nutrient-rich foods can provide the body with the necessary resources to cope with stress. Limiting the intake of stimulants such as caffeine and avoiding excessive alcohol consumption are additional dietary considerations for stress management.

Seeking professional support, such as counseling or therapy, is a proactive step for individuals experiencing persistent or overwhelming stress. Mental health professionals can provide guidance, coping strategies, and a supportive environment for addressing stressors and enhancing overall well-being.

In conclusion, stress management is integral to supporting prostate well-being, as chronic stress can contribute to the development and progression of prostate-related conditions. Implementing mindfulness practices, engaging in regular physical activity, fostering social connections, prioritizing sleep, and adopting a balanced diet are essential components of a comprehensive stress management strategy. By proactively addressing stress and incorporating these strategies into daily life, individuals can contribute to a healthier, more resilient response to stress and promote optimal prostate health throughout their lives.

The Influence of Mental Health on Physical Health

As an urologist, I am acutely aware of the intricate interplay between mental health and physical well-being, recognizing that a patient's psychological state can significantly influence their urological health. The impact of mental health on physical health is particularly pronounced in urology, where conditions ranging from erectile dysfunction and sexual health issues to urinary disorders can be intimately connected to an individual's mental and emotional state.

1. **Erectile Dysfunction and Mental Health:** Erectile dysfunction (ED) is a common concern among men, and mental health factors can play a crucial role in its onset and progression. Anxiety, depression, stress, and relationship issues can contribute to ED, creating a complex interrelationship between psychological and physiological factors. As an urologist, addressing the psychological aspects of ED is essential, often involving collaborative care with mental health professionals to ensure a holistic approach to treatment.

2. **Chronic Pelvic Pain Syndrome and Stress:** Chronic Pelvic Pain Syndrome (CPPS) is a challenging condition with multifaceted causes, and stress can be a significant exacerbating factor. Stress-induced muscular tension, heightened pain perception, and the bidirectional relationship between pain and mental health can contribute to the persistence of CPPS symptoms. Recognizing the

psychological dimensions of CPPS is crucial for comprehensive management, involving not only physical interventions but also strategies to alleviate stress and enhance coping mechanisms.

3. **Impact of Mental Health on Voiding Disorders:** Voiding disorders, such as overactive bladder or urinary incontinence, can be influenced by mental health factors. Anxiety, particularly related to concerns about accessing bathroom facilities or fear of embarrassment, can exacerbate symptoms. In such cases, addressing the emotional well-being of the patient becomes integral to the overall treatment plan. Behavioral and psychological interventions, in conjunction with urological treatments, aim to improve the patient's quality of life.

4. **Cancer Diagnosis and Mental Health:** A diagnosis of urological cancer, such as prostate or bladder cancer, can have profound psychological implications for patients. Understanding the emotional impact of a cancer diagnosis, including fear, anxiety, and depression, is essential in providing comprehensive care. As an urologist, working collaboratively with oncologists, psychologists, and support services becomes crucial to address both the physical aspects of cancer and the mental health challenges patients may face.

5. **Sexual Health and Relationship Dynamics:** Sexual health is a vital component of urological well-being, and mental health plays a central role in sexual function. Issues such as performance anxiety, body image concerns, and relationship dynamics can influence sexual satisfaction. Urologists need to

approach sexual health concerns with sensitivity, recognizing the interconnectedness of physical and mental aspects. Collaborative care involving sexual therapists or counselors may be warranted to address the broader context of sexual health.

Recognizing the influence of mental health on urological conditions requires a holistic approach that extends beyond traditional medical interventions. As an urologist, my role involves not only diagnosing and treating physical symptoms but also fostering an open dialogue about the emotional aspects of urological health. Collaborating with mental health professionals and integrating psychological support into the overall care plan is paramount to achieving optimal outcomes for patients.

In conclusion, the influence of mental health on physical health within the realm of urology is undeniable. Acknowledging the interconnectedness of physical and psychological well-being allows for a more comprehensive and patient-centered approach to urological care. By addressing mental health aspects, urologists contribute to a more holistic understanding of urological conditions and enhance the overall well-being of their patients.

Chapter 5: Medical Screenings and Checkups

Importance of Regular Checkups

Regular checkups are crucial for maintaining overall health and preventing potential health issues from escalating. As an urologist, I emphasize the importance of routine examinations, screenings, and health assessments to proactively manage urological conditions and contribute to a patient's overall well-being.

1. **Early Detection of Urological Conditions:** Regular checkups enable the early detection of urological conditions such as prostate cancer, kidney disorders, and urinary tract issues. Early diagnosis often allows for more effective treatment options and improved outcomes. For example, regular prostate screenings, including prostate-specific antigen (PSA) tests and digital rectal exams, play a critical role in detecting prostate cancer at an early, more treatable stage.

2. **Monitoring and Managing Chronic Conditions:** Patients with chronic urological conditions, such as benign prostatic hyperplasia (BPH) or chronic kidney disease, benefit significantly from regular checkups. These appointments provide an opportunity to monitor the progression of the condition, assess treatment efficacy, and make necessary adjustments to the management plan. Consistent monitoring is essential for maintaining

the optimal quality of life for individuals with chronic urological conditions.

3. **Prevention and Risk Assessment:** Regular checkups offer a platform for assessing individual health risks and implementing preventive measures. Urologists can evaluate a patient's risk factors for urological issues, such as family history, lifestyle factors, and age, and provide tailored advice on preventive strategies. This proactive approach is especially relevant for conditions like kidney stones or urinary tract infections, where lifestyle modifications can significantly reduce the risk of recurrence.

4. **Promoting Proactive Health Behavior:** Routine checkups serve as a foundation for fostering proactive health behavior. Engaging in regular health assessments encourages patients to take an active role in their well-being. Urologists can provide guidance on lifestyle modifications, such as maintaining a healthy diet, staying physically active, and avoiding tobacco and excessive alcohol consumption, which collectively contribute to urological health.

5. **Screening for Asymptomatic Conditions:** Some urological conditions may develop asymptomatically in their early stages. Regular checkups often involve screenings and diagnostic tests that can detect these conditions before symptoms manifest. For instance, imaging studies or urine tests may reveal kidney abnormalities or signs of bladder issues, allowing for timely intervention and prevention of complications.

6. **Patient Education and Awareness:** Checkup appointments serve as valuable opportunities for patient education and awareness. Urologists can provide information about urological health, symptoms to watch for, and the importance of seeking medical attention if any concerns arise. Educated patients are more likely to engage in preventive measures and make informed decisions about their health.

7. **Holistic Health Assessment:** Regular checkups offer a holistic assessment of an individual's health beyond specific urological concerns. Urologists can collaborate with other healthcare providers to ensure comprehensive care, addressing the interconnectedness of various aspects of health. For example, understanding the influence of lifestyle factors, mental health, and chronic conditions on urological health contributes to a more integrated and patient-centered approach.

In conclusion, regular checkups are instrumental in promoting urological health and overall well-being. As an urologist, I encourage patients to prioritize preventive care, attend routine examinations, and actively engage in their health management. Proactive healthcare, including regular checkups, not only facilitates early detection and intervention but also empowers individuals to make informed choices that support their long-term urological and overall health.

Understanding Prostate-Specific Antigen (PSA) Tests

As an urologist, understanding the intricacies of Prostate-Specific Antigen (PSA) tests is essential for both accurate diagnosis and informed patient discussions. PSA is a protein produced by the prostate gland, and its levels in the blood can be indicative of various prostate conditions, including prostate cancer. The PSA test is a valuable tool in urology, but its interpretation requires a nuanced approach. Elevated PSA levels can prompt further investigation, but it's crucial to recognize that a high PSA reading doesn't definitively diagnose prostate cancer. Instead, it raises a flag, necessitating additional assessments such as digital rectal exams (DRE) and imaging studies to provide a comprehensive evaluation. Conversely, normal PSA levels do not guarantee the absence of prostate cancer. Understanding the factors influencing PSA levels is imperative; age, prostate size, inflammation, and recent activities like ejaculation or cycling can impact readings. Engaging patients in open dialogues about the benefits and limitations of PSA testing is integral to shared decision-making. It allows urologists to guide patients through personalized risk assessments, considering individual health history, preferences, and potential consequences of further diagnostic interventions. In this collaborative approach, the PSA test becomes a valuable component in a broader strategy aimed at accurate diagnosis, timely intervention, and informed patient care.

The PSA test's primary objective is to detect elevated levels of the prostate-specific antigen, a protein produced by the prostate gland. While the test has been instrumental in identifying potential prostate issues, particularly prostate cancer, its interpretation requires a nuanced understanding. Elevated PSA levels can indicate several conditions, not exclusively cancer, such as benign prostatic hyperplasia (BPH) or prostatitis, an inflammation of the prostate. Therefore, the PSA test is not a definitive diagnostic tool but rather a crucial screening method that necessitates further evaluation. It's important for urologists to convey this nuance to patients, ensuring they comprehend that an elevated PSA reading does not equate to a cancer diagnosis. A comprehensive assessment, including a digital rectal exam (DRE) and additional imaging studies, is essential to provide a more accurate picture of the patient's prostate health. Conversely, normal PSA levels do not entirely rule out the possibility of prostate cancer. Urologists must navigate these complexities with patients, fostering open discussions about the benefits and limitations of PSA testing, while considering individual factors such as age, health history, and personal preferences. This patient-centered approach allows for shared decision-making, empowering individuals to actively participate in their healthcare journey.

Understanding the factors influencing PSA levels is paramount for accurate interpretation and subsequent decision-making. Age plays a significant role, as PSA levels tend to rise gradually with age. However, defining a specific PSA threshold for further investigation is challenging, and guidelines often vary. Prostate size, influenced by factors like BPH, can impact PSA readings; larger prostates typically yield higher PSA levels. Inflammation within the prostate, as seen in prostatitis, can also elevate PSA levels. Additionally, recent activities such as ejaculation or certain exercises like cycling can temporarily increase PSA levels. Urologists must consider these variables when assessing

PSA results to avoid unnecessary concern or oversight. Communicating these nuances to patients is vital, fostering an understanding that PSA levels are influenced by a spectrum of factors, and elevated readings prompt a comprehensive evaluation rather than an immediate cancer diagnosis.

Open and transparent communication with patients about the benefits and limitations of PSA testing is integral to informed decision-making. Engaging patients in discussions about their individual risk factors, preferences, and potential consequences of further diagnostic interventions empowers them to actively participate in their healthcare decisions. For some, the PSA test may be a valuable tool in monitoring prostate health, while others may prioritize avoiding potential overdiagnosis and overtreatment. Urologists must guide patients through this decision-making process, providing the necessary information to make informed choices aligned with their values and health priorities. Shared decision-making transforms the PSA test from a standalone screening tool into a collaborative element of a broader strategy focused on personalized care and optimal patient outcomes.

Moreover, in the context of prostate cancer diagnosis and management, the PSA test serves as a crucial baseline metric for tracking changes over time. Serial PSA measurements, when interpreted judiciously, contribute to the monitoring of disease progression and response to treatment. In cases where prostate cancer is diagnosed, the PSA test becomes an essential tool for risk stratification and ongoing surveillance. Understanding the kinetics of PSA changes, including the rate of increase (PSA velocity) and the doubling time, allows urologists to tailor treatment plans and interventions based on the unique characteristics of the individual's cancer. This nuanced approach to PSA monitoring exemplifies its multifaceted role in urological care, extending beyond initial screening to guide ongoing management decisions for patients with prostate cancer.

In conclusion, as an urologist, navigating the complexities of PSA testing involves recognizing its role as a valuable screening tool and understanding its limitations. Engaging in open discussions with patients about the nuances of PSA interpretation, individual risk factors, and the potential consequences of further diagnostic interventions is essential for informed decision-making. The PSA test, when integrated into a broader strategy of personalized care, facilitates accurate diagnosis, timely intervention, and ongoing monitoring, contributing to optimal urological health outcomes for patients.

Chapter 6: Preventive Measures and Habits

Promoting Prostate Health Through Healthy Habits

Promoting prostate health through healthy habits is a proactive and empowering approach to safeguarding one's well-being. Incorporating lifestyle choices that support a healthy prostate not only mitigates the risk of certain conditions but also contributes to overall urological and general health. Here, we delve into a comprehensive exploration of the various healthy habits that play a pivotal role in promoting prostate health.

1. Balanced Diet: At the core of promoting prostate health is maintaining a balanced and nutrient-rich diet. Fruits and vegetables, particularly those rich in antioxidants like tomatoes, berries, and leafy greens, provide essential vitamins and minerals. Cruciferous vegetables such as broccoli and cauliflower contain compounds that may have protective effects. Additionally, incorporating foods with omega-3 fatty acids, like fatty fish (salmon, mackerel), walnuts, and flaxseeds, contributes to overall anti-inflammatory benefits that may impact prostate health positively.

2. Prostate-Friendly Foods: Specific foods are recognized for their potential benefits to prostate health. Tomatoes, for example, contain lycopene, a potent antioxidant associated with a lower risk of prostate cancer. Selenium-rich foods, including Brazil nuts, fish, and turkey, are essential for maintaining prostate health. Green tea, known for its polyphenolic compounds, has been studied for its potential anti-cancer properties. Integrating these prostate-friendly foods into the diet provides a targeted approach to supporting the health of this vital organ.

3. Hydration: Staying well-hydrated is crucial for overall health, and it plays a role in prostate health as well. Adequate hydration supports urinary function, helping to flush toxins and waste products from the body. Water is the ideal beverage choice, and individuals are encouraged to limit the intake of caffeinated and alcoholic beverages, which can contribute to dehydration.

4. Regular Exercise: Engaging in regular physical activity is a cornerstone of promoting prostate health. Exercise has been linked to a lower risk of prostate cancer and can aid in the management of conditions such as benign prostatic hyperplasia (BPH). Both aerobic exercises, like brisk walking or jogging, and strength training contribute to overall fitness and may have specific benefits for prostate health. Incorporating at least 150 minutes of moderate-intensity exercise per week is recommended.

5. Maintaining a Healthy Weight: Maintaining a healthy weight is intricately linked to prostate health. Obesity is associated with an increased risk of prostate cancer and other urological conditions. Adopting a balanced diet and engaging in regular physical activity are key components of weight management. Lifestyle changes that contribute to weight loss can have positive effects on both prostate health and overall well-being.

6. Limiting Red and Processed Meats: Dietary choices play a crucial role in prostate health, and limiting the intake of red and processed meats is advisable. High consumption of red and processed meats has been associated with an increased risk of prostate cancer. Choosing lean protein sources such as poultry, fish, beans, and legumes is a prudent dietary decision that aligns with promoting prostate health.

7. Moderate Calcium Intake: Calcium is an essential mineral, but excessive intake, primarily through supplements, has been linked to an increased risk of prostate cancer. Maintaining a moderate and balanced intake of calcium through dietary sources, such as dairy products, leafy greens, and fortified foods, is advisable. It's essential to consult with healthcare professionals before considering calcium supplements.

8. Vitamin D: Adequate vitamin D levels are associated with a lower risk of aggressive prostate cancer. Sun exposure is a natural source of vitamin D, and incorporating foods like fatty fish, egg yolks, and fortified products can contribute to sufficient intake. In some cases, supplements may be recommended, but it's crucial to determine individual needs through consultation with healthcare providers.

9. Limiting Alcohol Consumption: Excessive alcohol consumption has been linked to an increased risk of prostate cancer. Moderation is key, and limiting alcohol intake to moderate levels—defined as up to one drink per day for men—is advisable. This approach aligns with overall health guidelines and contributes to prostate health.

10. Regular Health Checkups: Proactive engagement with healthcare through regular checkups is vital for promoting prostate health. Routine screenings, such as the prostate-specific antigen (PSA) test and digital rectal examination (DRE), enable the early detection of potential issues. These screenings are particularly relevant for individuals with risk factors such as age, family history, or specific ethnic backgrounds.

11. Stress Management: Chronic stress can impact overall health, including prostate health. Incorporating stress management techniques, such as mindfulness meditation, deep breathing exercises, or regular relaxation practices, contributes to a holistic approach to well-being. Managing stress is not only beneficial for mental health but may also have positive effects on prostate health.

12. No Smoking: Smoking is associated with an increased risk of developing aggressive forms of prostate cancer. Quitting smoking is a crucial step toward promoting prostate health and overall longevity. Smoking cessation has numerous health benefits and contributes to a healthier lifestyle.

In conclusion, promoting prostate health through healthy habits involves a comprehensive and integrative approach. Adopting a balanced diet, engaging in regular exercise, maintaining a healthy weight, and making informed lifestyle choices contribute to overall urological well-being. It's essential to tailor these habits to individual needs, considering factors such as age, existing health conditions, and genetic predispositions.

Supplements and Their Role

As a urologist, the topic of supplements and their role in promoting urological health is multifaceted. While supplements can offer potential benefits, it's crucial for individuals to approach their use with an informed perspective and, when necessary, under the guidance of healthcare professionals. Certain supplements have garnered attention for their possible positive impact on prostate health. For instance, saw palmetto, a plant extract, has been explored for its potential in managing benign prostatic hyperplasia (BPH), a common condition in aging men. Some studies suggest that saw palmetto may alleviate BPH symptoms, but conclusive evidence is still lacking, and its efficacy can vary among individuals. Additionally, beta-sitosterol, a plant-derived sterol, has been studied for its potential to improve urinary symptoms associated with BPH. However, the overall scientific consensus on its effectiveness remains inconclusive. It's crucial for patients to consult with their urologists before incorporating such supplements into their routine, as individual responses can vary, and potential interactions with medications need to be considered.

Omega-3 fatty acids, commonly found in fish oil supplements, have been studied for their anti-inflammatory properties, and some research suggests a potential link between omega-3 intake and a lower risk of prostate cancer. While this association is intriguing, more robust clinical evidence is needed to establish definitive recommendations. Furthermore, vitamin D has gained attention for its potential role in prostate health. Adequate vitamin D levels are associated with a lower risk of aggressive prostate cancer, and supplementation may be beneficial for individuals with insufficient vitamin D levels. However, excessive vitamin D intake can have adverse effects, emphasizing the importance of personalized recommendations based on individual health profiles.

Antioxidant supplements, including vitamin E and selenium, have been explored for their potential protective effects against prostate cancer. However, large-scale clinical trials, such as the SELECT trial, did not conclusively demonstrate a significant reduction in prostate cancer risk with vitamin E and selenium supplementation. In fact, excessive intake of these supplements may have adverse effects. As an urologist, my approach is to advocate for obtaining essential nutrients through a well-balanced diet rather than relying solely on supplements. Fruits, vegetables, and whole grains provide a spectrum of vitamins, minerals, and antioxidants that contribute to overall health and may indirectly support urological well-being.

While there is ongoing research on the potential benefits of supplements for urological health, it's essential to approach these findings with a level of caution. The field of supplements and their impact on specific urological conditions is dynamic, and recommendations may evolve as more evidence becomes available. As healthcare professionals, urologists play a vital role in guiding patients through the complexities of supplement use. It's important for patients to disclose their supplement intake during medical consultations, as certain supplements may interact with medications or impact urological conditions.

Furthermore, urologists can provide evidence-based recommendations tailored to individual health needs. For instance, individuals at risk of kidney stones may benefit from increased fluid intake and dietary modifications rather than relying solely on supplements. Additionally, lifestyle factors such as maintaining a healthy weight, engaging in regular physical activity, and avoiding tobacco and excessive alcohol consumption play pivotal roles in urological health and should not be overshadowed by a reliance on supplements.

In conclusion, while supplements may offer potential benefits for urological health, their use should be approached judiciously, considering individual health profiles and potential interactions with medications. Urologists can provide personalized guidance based on the latest scientific evidence, emphasizing the importance of a well-balanced diet, lifestyle modifications, and informed decision-making. As the field of supplements and urological health continues to evolve, collaborative discussions between healthcare professionals and patients remain paramount in ensuring optimal urological well-being.

Chapter 7: Common Prostate Conditions

Exploring Conditions such as BPH and Prostatitis

As a practicing urologist, I understand the significance of addressing conditions such as Benign Prostatic Hyperplasia (BPH) and Prostatitis with the utmost care and precision. These urological conditions, while distinct in their nature, share the potential to impact a patient's quality of life, and it is essential to approach them with a comprehensive understanding of their implications and available medical interventions.

1. **Benign Prostatic Hyperplasia (BPH):** Benign Prostatic Hyperplasia, commonly referred to as BPH, is a non-cancerous enlargement of the prostate gland that can lead to urinary symptoms. As a urologist, my primary goal is to provide a thorough assessment to understand the extent of your condition. Diagnostic measures typically include a detailed medical history, a physical examination, and potentially additional tests such as a prostate-specific antigen (PSA) test or urinalysis. Treatment options for BPH range from lifestyle modifications to medications and, in some cases, surgical interventions. It is crucial to tailor the approach based on the severity of symptoms, impact on daily life, and individual health considerations. I recommend maintaining open communication throughout this process to ensure that your concerns are addressed, and together, we

can develop a personalized and effective management plan.

2. **Prostatitis:** Prostatitis refers to the inflammation of the prostate gland, a condition that can manifest in various forms, including acute or chronic bacterial prostatitis, chronic pelvic pain syndrome, and asymptomatic inflammatory prostatitis. Accurate diagnosis is pivotal, and my approach as a urologist involves a meticulous evaluation, which may include a detailed medical history, a physical examination, and laboratory tests. The choice of treatment depends on the specific type of prostatitis diagnosed. Antibiotics may be prescribed for bacterial prostatitis, while other forms may require a combination of medications and lifestyle modifications. In chronic cases, a multidisciplinary approach involving physical therapy and stress management techniques may be recommended. Throughout the treatment process, I emphasize the importance of regular follow-up appointments to monitor progress and adjust the management plan as needed.

In both cases, BPH and Prostatitis, it is imperative to prioritize proactive measures for maintaining urological health. Lifestyle modifications, including maintaining a balanced diet, staying physically active, and managing stress, can contribute significantly to overall well-being. As your urologist, my commitment is to provide comprehensive care, addressing not only the immediate symptoms but also the underlying factors that contribute to the conditions. I encourage open communication, ensuring that you are informed about your condition, involved in decision-making, and comfortable discussing any concerns that may arise during the course of diagnosis and treatment.

Please be advised that the information provided here is for general understanding, and individual cases may vary. It is essential to schedule an in-person consultation for a detailed assessment, accurate diagnosis, and personalized medical advice based on your specific health profile. I look forward to working collaboratively to address your urological concerns and contribute to your overall well-being.

Symptoms, Treatment Options, and Management

As a dedicated urologist, addressing symptoms, treatment options, and management strategies for urological conditions is a critical aspect of my medical practice. Patients experiencing symptoms related to urological issues require a comprehensive understanding of their condition, effective treatment modalities, and tailored management plans to ensure optimal outcomes.

Symptoms Evaluation: When patients present with urological symptoms, a meticulous evaluation is paramount. These symptoms may include urinary changes, pelvic pain, sexual dysfunction, or abnormalities detected during routine screenings. As a urologist, my initial approach involves a thorough medical history assessment and a detailed discussion of your symptoms. This is complemented by a physical examination, and, if necessary, diagnostic tests such as imaging studies, urine analyses, or specialized urodynamic assessments. Understanding the specific nature and severity of symptoms is crucial in formulating an accurate diagnosis and determining the most appropriate course of action.

Treatment Options: The array of treatment options available for urological conditions reflects the diverse nature of these issues. Personalizing treatment plans is a key principle in my practice, ensuring that each patient receives care tailored to their unique health profile and individual needs.

1. **Medication:** Prescription medications often play a pivotal role in managing urological conditions. For

instance, in cases of Benign Prostatic Hyperplasia (BPH), medications such as alpha-blockers or 5-alpha reductase inhibitors may be prescribed to alleviate urinary symptoms. Similarly, antibiotics are frequently employed for bacterial prostatitis. In the realm of erectile dysfunction, phosphodiesterase type 5 (PDE5) inhibitors may be recommended.

2. **Minimally Invasive Procedures:** In certain scenarios, minimally invasive procedures may offer effective solutions. For BPH, procedures like transurethral resection of the prostate (TURP) or laser therapy can provide relief from obstructive symptoms. Urologists may also employ minimally invasive techniques for kidney stone removal or addressing certain forms of urinary incontinence.

3. **Surgical Interventions:** Surgical interventions become relevant in cases where conservative measures prove insufficient. Procedures such as prostatectomy may be considered for prostate cancer, and surgical approaches vary based on the specific characteristics of the condition.

4. **Lifestyle Modifications:** Lifestyle plays a significant role in managing urological conditions. Dietary adjustments, regular exercise, and stress management techniques can contribute to overall well-being and positively impact symptoms. For instance, dietary modifications may be recommended for conditions like kidney stones, emphasizing increased fluid intake and reduced sodium consumption.

Management Strategies: Beyond the immediate treatment phase, effective management strategies are pivotal for long-term urological health. Regular follow-up appointments allow for ongoing monitoring, ensuring that any changes in symptoms or treatment efficacy are promptly addressed. This continuous evaluation is particularly crucial for chronic conditions such as chronic prostatitis or conditions requiring long-term medication management.

Patient education is integral to the management process. Ensuring that patients are well-informed about their condition, treatment options, and potential side effects empowers them to actively participate in their healthcare journey. I encourage open communication during appointments, providing a platform for patients to express concerns, ask questions, and collaborate in decision-making.

Psychosocial support is an often underestimated but essential component of urological care. Conditions like erectile dysfunction or urinary incontinence can have significant psychological impacts. Offering resources, counseling, or referrals to specialists in sexual health or mental health when necessary contributes to a holistic approach in managing these aspects of urological conditions.

In conclusion, addressing symptoms, exploring treatment options, and implementing effective management strategies form the cornerstone of urological care. As a urologist, my commitment is to provide patient-centered care, leveraging evidence-based approaches, and fostering open communication. By tailoring treatment plans to individual needs and considering the broader context of each patient's health, I aim to contribute to not only symptom relief but also the overall well-being of individuals experiencing urological conditions.

Chapter 8: Treatment and Intervention

Available Treatment Options

As a dedicated urologist, navigating the spectrum of available treatment options for various urological conditions is integral to providing comprehensive and effective care. The diverse nature of urological issues necessitates a nuanced approach, considering factors such as the specific condition, its severity, and individual patient characteristics.

1. Medications: Prescription medications often serve as a cornerstone in the management of urological conditions. For instance, alpha-blockers and 5-alpha reductase inhibitors are commonly prescribed to alleviate urinary symptoms associated with Benign Prostatic Hyperplasia (BPH). Antibiotics play a crucial role in treating bacterial prostatitis, while medications like phosphodiesterase type 5 (PDE5) inhibitors are employed for erectile dysfunction. Selective serotonin and norepinephrine reuptake inhibitors (SSRIs and SNRIs) may be recommended for certain cases of chronic pelvic pain syndrome.

2. Minimally Invasive Procedures: Minimally invasive procedures offer effective solutions with reduced recovery times. Urologists may employ procedures such as transurethral resection of the prostate (TURP) or laser therapy for BPH, providing relief from obstructive symptoms. Procedures like extracorporeal shock wave lithotripsy (ESWL) are utilized for kidney stones, breaking them into smaller fragments for easier passage. Additionally, minimally invasive approaches for urinary incontinence, such as the insertion of slings or bulking agents, can provide significant improvement in symptoms.

3. Surgical Interventions: Surgical interventions become relevant when more conservative measures prove inadequate. For prostate cancer, procedures like radical prostatectomy or robotic-assisted laparoscopic prostatectomy may be recommended. Similarly, surgical interventions are considered for conditions such as bladder or kidney cancer, addressing the specific characteristics and staging of the disease.

4. Lifestyle Modifications: Lifestyle modifications play a pivotal role in managing urological conditions. Dietary adjustments, including increased fluid intake for kidney stone prevention or dietary changes for individuals with interstitial cystitis, can contribute to symptom relief. Regular exercise and stress management techniques are also emphasized to enhance overall well-being and positively impact urological health.

5. Behavioral Therapies: Behavioral therapies are integral in managing conditions such as urinary incontinence. Pelvic floor exercises, bladder training, and biofeedback techniques are commonly employed to improve bladder control and alleviate symptoms. These approaches aim to enhance the coordination of pelvic floor muscles and improve overall bladder function.

6. Implantable Devices: In some cases, implantable devices offer viable treatment options. For erectile dysfunction, penile implants may be considered when other interventions are not effective. Similarly, artificial urinary sphincters or sacral neuromodulation devices are utilized in the management of urinary incontinence.

7. Chemotherapy and Radiation Therapy: In the context of urological cancers, such as bladder or prostate cancer, chemotherapy and radiation therapy are vital treatment modalities. These approaches are tailored to the specific characteristics of the cancer, its stage, and the overall health of the patient. The goal is to target and eliminate cancer cells while minimizing damage to healthy surrounding tissues.

8. Follow-Up and Monitoring: Continuous follow-up and monitoring are essential components of urological care. Regular appointments allow for ongoing assessment of treatment efficacy, adjustment of management plans as needed, and the early detection of any potential complications or recurrent symptoms. Patient engagement in the follow-up process is encouraged, fostering a collaborative approach to long-term urological health.

In conclusion, the spectrum of available treatment options for urological conditions reflects the dynamic and evolving nature of urological care. As a urologist, my commitment is to navigate this landscape judiciously, tailoring treatment plans to individual needs, and prioritizing patient-centered care. By considering the comprehensive range of available interventions and incorporating evidence-based approaches, I aim to contribute to the optimal management and well-being of individuals facing urological challenges.

Navigating Decision-Making with Healthcare Professionals

Navigating decision-making in the realm of urological health is a collaborative journey between healthcare professionals, such as urologists, and patients. Let's delve into a hypothetical scenario to illustrate this intricate process. Consider Mr. Johnson, a patient presenting with symptoms suggestive of a prostate condition. As a urologist, my initial interaction with Mr. Johnson involves a comprehensive evaluation, including a detailed medical history, physical examination, and relevant diagnostic tests. The nuanced understanding of Mr. Johnson's health profile forms the foundation for informed decision-making.

Upon confirming a diagnosis of Benign Prostatic Hyperplasia (BPH), we embark on a shared exploration of treatment options. Here, the collaborative decision-making process unfolds through several key steps.

1. Patient Education: The first pillar of collaborative decision-making is patient education. I take the time to elucidate the nature of BPH, its implications, and the available treatment modalities. By providing Mr. Johnson with comprehensive information about the condition, its progression, and potential treatment outcomes, I empower him to actively participate in the decision-making process.

2. Discussion of Treatment Options: In a conversational and accessible manner, we discuss the array of treatment options tailored to Mr. Johnson's specific health profile. Medications, minimally invasive procedures like transurethral resection of the prostate (TURP), and lifestyle modifications all come under scrutiny. Each option is presented with its potential benefits, risks, and expected outcomes. This dialogue ensures that Mr. Johnson gains a nuanced understanding of the choices before him.

3. Shared Decision-Making: With a foundation of knowledge in place, the decision-making process shifts towards collaboration. Mr. Johnson's preferences, lifestyle, and personal priorities become integral factors. We engage in a candid discussion about his expectations, concerns, and the impact of each treatment option on his daily life. Shared decision-making, in this context, is not a one-size-fits-all approach but rather a personalized exploration of what aligns best with Mr. Johnson's values and health goals.

4. Informed Consent: In tandem with shared decision-making, the principle of informed consent is upheld. I ensure that Mr. Johnson comprehensively understands the potential benefits and risks associated with each treatment option. This includes a discussion about potential side effects, the likelihood of success, and any long-term considerations. Mr. Johnson's active involvement in this process is essential, emphasizing autonomy and mutual understanding.

5. Multidisciplinary Collaboration: The decision-making journey extends beyond the urologist's office. In cases where additional expertise is warranted, collaboration with other healthcare professionals comes to the forefront. This may involve consultations with primary care physicians, pharmacists, or specialists in related fields. A multidisciplinary approach ensures that Mr. Johnson receives holistic and well-rounded care, addressing not only the immediate urological concerns but also considering the broader context of his health.

6. Ongoing Communication: The decision-making process doesn't conclude with the initiation of treatment. Ongoing communication is a cornerstone of effective healthcare. Regular follow-up appointments provide a platform for Mr. Johnson to share his experiences, discuss any emerging concerns, and assess the progress of the chosen treatment plan. This iterative communication allows for adjustments to be made based on Mr. Johnson's response to treatment and any evolving health considerations.

7. Integration of Patient Preferences: Patient preferences are central to the decision-making process. Mr. Johnson's input shapes the trajectory of his care, acknowledging that the chosen treatment plan aligns with his values and lifestyle. Whether opting for a medication regimen that fits seamlessly into his routine or choosing a procedure that aligns with his expectations, the integration of patient preferences ensures a more patient-centric and satisfactory healthcare experience.

In this hypothetical scenario, the collaborative decision-making process culminates in a treatment plan that aligns with Mr. Johnson's preferences, addresses his urological concerns, and considers his overall well-being. By fostering open communication, providing comprehensive education, and integrating patient preferences, the urologist-patient partnership becomes a dynamic force in navigating the complexities of prostate health.

The success of this collaborative approach extends beyond the immediate treatment phase. It lays the groundwork for a sustained and trusting relationship between Mr. Johnson and his healthcare team. Through ongoing communication, periodic assessments, and a commitment to patient-centered care, the urologist serves not only as a medical guide but as a partner in Mr. Johnson's journey toward optimal urological health.

Chapter 9: Emotional Well-Being

Coping with Prostate Health Challenges

Coping with prostate health challenges involves a multifaceted approach that encompasses physical, emotional, and psychological dimensions. Let's delve into a comprehensive discussion on navigating the complexities of prostate health challenges, offering insights into coping strategies and considerations.

Physical Coping Strategies:

1. **Treatment Adherence:** A cornerstone of physical coping is adherence to the prescribed treatment plan. Whether it involves medication regimens, lifestyle modifications, or surgical interventions, consistent adherence is paramount. Patients are encouraged to maintain open communication with their healthcare providers, reporting any side effects, concerns, or changes in symptoms promptly.

2. **Lifestyle Modifications:** Implementing lifestyle changes can significantly contribute to physical well-being. Dietary modifications, such as adopting a prostate-friendly diet rich in antioxidants, omega-3 fatty acids, and nutrients, can positively impact prostate health. Regular exercise, tailored to individual capabilities, not only promotes overall health but also aids in managing specific conditions like benign prostatic hyperplasia (BPH) or erectile dysfunction.

3. **Pelvic Floor Exercises:** For individuals dealing with conditions affecting the pelvic region, such as urinary incontinence or erectile dysfunction, pelvic floor exercises can be beneficial. These exercises, including Kegel exercises, help strengthen the pelvic floor muscles, contributing to improved bladder control and sexual function.

4. **Pain Management Techniques:** Prostate health challenges may be accompanied by pain or discomfort. Employing pain management techniques, ranging from over-the-counter medications to prescribed pain relievers, can enhance physical comfort. Integrative approaches like acupuncture or physical therapy may also be explored under the guidance of healthcare professionals.

5. **Regular Medical Checkups:** Ongoing monitoring through regular medical checkups is crucial for managing prostate health challenges. These checkups facilitate the early detection of any changes in symptoms, treatment efficacy, or potential complications. Consistent follow-up appointments with healthcare providers ensure a proactive and preventive approach to urological well-being.

Emotional Coping Strategies:

1. **Patient Education:** Understanding one's condition is a powerful tool for emotional coping. Patient education, facilitated by healthcare professionals, provides individuals with the knowledge needed to comprehend the nature of their prostate health challenges, potential treatment options, and expected

outcomes. Informed patients are better equipped to navigate the emotional aspects of their health journey.

2. **Peer Support and Support Groups:** Connecting with peers who share similar experiences can provide invaluable emotional support. Support groups for prostate health challenges create a platform for individuals to share their journeys, exchange coping strategies, and foster a sense of community. Peer support helps combat feelings of isolation and promotes a shared understanding of the emotional nuances associated with urological conditions.

3. **Professional Counseling:** Emotional well-being is intricately linked to mental health. Seeking professional counseling or therapy can be instrumental in navigating the emotional impact of prostate health challenges. Counseling sessions provide a safe space to express concerns, manage stress, and develop coping mechanisms tailored to individual needs.

4. **Open Communication with Loved Ones:** Engaging in open communication with loved ones is pivotal for emotional coping. Sharing one's experiences, concerns, and triumphs with a support network promotes a sense of understanding and empathy. Loved ones can play a vital role in offering emotional support and creating a conducive environment for healing.

5. **Mind-Body Practices:** Mind-body practices, including mindfulness meditation, deep breathing exercises, and yoga, offer tools for emotional coping.

These practices promote relaxation, reduce stress, and contribute to an overall sense of well-being. Integrating mind-body techniques into daily routines empowers individuals to manage the emotional toll of prostate health challenges.

Psychological Coping Strategies:

1. **Mindful Acceptance:** Accepting the reality of a prostate health challenge is an essential psychological coping strategy. Mindful acceptance involves acknowledging the condition, understanding its implications, and fostering resilience to navigate the journey ahead. This mindset lays the foundation for proactive engagement with treatment and lifestyle adjustments.

2. **Goal Setting and Positive Visualization:** Setting realistic goals and visualizing positive outcomes can positively impact psychological well-being. Establishing achievable milestones, whether related to treatment adherence, lifestyle changes, or overall health improvement, instills a sense of purpose and optimism. Positive visualization reinforces the belief in one's ability to overcome challenges.

3. **Resilience Building:** Building resilience involves cultivating adaptive coping mechanisms in the face of adversity. Psychologically resilient individuals are better equipped to navigate setbacks, embrace change, and maintain a positive outlook. Strategies for resilience building may include developing a strong support system, practicing self-compassion, and fostering a growth mindset.

4. **Cognitive-Behavioral Techniques:** Cognitive-behavioral techniques, guided by mental health professionals, can be effective in managing psychological distress. These techniques address thought patterns, emotions, and behaviors, empowering individuals to reframe negative perceptions, manage stress, and enhance psychological resilience.

5. **Empowerment through Information:** Empowerment through information involves actively seeking knowledge about one's condition and participating in decision-making processes. Informed individuals feel a sense of control over their health journey, reducing feelings of helplessness. Healthcare providers play a crucial role in facilitating this empowerment by offering transparent and comprehensive information.

In conclusion, coping with prostate health challenges is a holistic endeavor that encompasses physical, emotional, and psychological dimensions. By integrating lifestyle modifications, seeking emotional support, and adopting resilient mindsets, individuals can navigate their health journeys with a sense of empowerment and well-being. Healthcare professionals, including urologists, play a pivotal role in guiding patients through these multifaceted coping strategies, fostering a collaborative approach to urological care.

Building a Support System

Building a robust support system is instrumental in navigating life's challenges, and this holds particularly true for individuals facing prostate health issues. Establishing a network of support goes beyond the realms of emotional comfort; it becomes a pillar of strength that enhances overall well-being. In the context of prostate health challenges, this support system plays a pivotal role in fostering resilience, encouraging adherence to treatment plans, and promoting a positive outlook on the journey ahead.

1. Family and Friends: The foundation of any support system often lies within the familial and friendship circles. Loved ones, including family members and close friends, provide an essential network that offers emotional understanding, encouragement, and companionship. They serve as pillars of strength during medical appointments, treatments, and the overall management of prostate health challenges.

2. Peer Support Groups: Connecting with individuals who share similar experiences forms a unique layer of support. Peer support groups specifically tailored for those dealing with prostate health challenges offer a space for shared understanding and empathy. Members of these groups exchange insights, coping strategies, and practical tips, fostering a sense of camaraderie that combats feelings of isolation.

3. Healthcare Professionals: The relationship between individuals facing prostate health challenges and their healthcare providers forms a critical component of the support system. Open communication with urologists, nurses, and other healthcare professionals establishes a foundation of trust. These professionals not only guide patients through medical decisions but also offer valuable information and resources, empowering individuals to actively participate in their care.

4. Counselors and Therapists: Emotional well-being is intricately connected to mental health, and seeking the expertise of counselors or therapists can be transformative. These professionals provide a safe space for individuals to express their fears, anxieties, and emotional challenges. Through counseling, individuals can develop coping strategies, manage stress, and build resilience in the face of prostate health challenges.

5. Community Resources: Community resources, including local organizations, support networks, and educational programs, contribute to a well-rounded support system. These resources offer a wealth of information, organize awareness events, and facilitate connections with others facing similar challenges. Engaging with community resources expands the support network beyond personal relationships, creating a broader sense of belonging.

6. Online Communities: In the digital age, online communities play a significant role in building support systems. Virtual forums, social media groups, and dedicated platforms connect individuals from diverse locations, allowing for the exchange of experiences and insights. Online communities offer accessible and immediate support, particularly for those who may face geographical or mobility constraints.

7. Caregivers: For individuals dealing with prostate health challenges, caregivers assume a crucial role within the support system. Whether it's a spouse, family member, or hired caregiver, their assistance in daily activities, emotional encouragement, and advocacy during medical appointments contribute significantly to the overall well-being of the individual.

8. Educational Programs: Participating in educational programs focused on prostate health not only enhances knowledge but also fosters connections with others on a similar journey. Workshops, seminars, and webinars provide opportunities for individuals to learn, ask questions, and share experiences, creating a supportive environment grounded in understanding.

In essence, building a support system for those facing prostate health challenges is about weaving a tapestry of interconnected relationships. This network becomes a source of strength during moments of uncertainty, a repository of shared wisdom, and a collective force that empowers individuals to face their health challenges with resilience and optimism. As urologists and healthcare professionals, part of our role is to encourage patients to recognize the importance of this support system and facilitate connections that contribute to their overall well-being.

Chapter 10: Future Trends and Research

Advances in Prostate Health Research

Advances in prostate health research represent a dynamic frontier in understanding, preventing, and treating various conditions affecting this vital organ. Cutting-edge investigations are reshaping our comprehension of prostate health, encompassing a spectrum of areas from cancer prevention to innovative treatment modalities.

1. Early Detection and Screening: Research in prostate health has witnessed significant strides in refining early detection methods. The traditional prostate-specific antigen (PSA) test, while valuable, is being complemented by novel approaches that enhance specificity and reduce false positives. Biomarker discovery, genetic profiling, and advanced imaging technologies, such as multiparametric magnetic resonance imaging (mpMRI), are at the forefront. These innovations aim to improve the accuracy of prostate cancer diagnosis, enabling more precise risk stratification and personalized treatment strategies.

2. Precision Medicine and Genomic Research: The era of precision medicine is influencing prostate health research profoundly. Genomic studies are unraveling the intricate molecular landscape of prostate cancer, identifying key genetic mutations and variations. This knowledge is paving the way for targeted therapies that address specific genomic alterations. Tailoring treatment plans based on the individual genetic makeup of the patient holds immense promise in optimizing outcomes and minimizing side effects.

3. Immunotherapy Breakthroughs: Immunotherapy has emerged as a groundbreaking avenue in prostate health research, particularly in the context of advanced prostate cancer. Approaches such as immune checkpoint inhibitors and therapeutic cancer vaccines are undergoing rigorous investigation. These strategies aim to harness the body's immune system to target and eliminate cancer cells selectively. Immunotherapy, with its potential for durable responses, represents a paradigm shift in the treatment landscape for certain prostate cancers.

4. Lifestyle and Environmental Influences: Contemporary research is increasingly exploring the interplay between lifestyle factors, environmental exposures, and prostate health. Investigations delve into the impact of diet, physical activity, and environmental toxins on prostate cancer risk. Understanding these influences at a molecular level provides insights into potential preventive measures and lifestyle modifications that may mitigate the risk of prostate cancer development.

5. Artificial Intelligence in Diagnosis and Risk Stratification: The integration of artificial intelligence (AI) in prostate health research is revolutionizing diagnostic capabilities. AI algorithms, trained on vast datasets of medical imaging and clinical information, demonstrate remarkable accuracy in detecting and characterizing prostate lesions. These technologies not only expedite diagnosis but also contribute to more informed decision-making in treatment planning and risk stratification.

6. Advancements in Minimally Invasive Treatments:
Treatment modalities for prostate conditions have seen notable advancements, particularly in the realm of minimally invasive interventions. Robotic-assisted surgeries, such as robot-assisted laparoscopic prostatectomy, have become standard in the surgical management of prostate cancer. These techniques offer enhanced precision, reduced recovery times, and improved postoperative outcomes, shaping the landscape of prostate surgery.

7. Prostate Cancer Risk Prediction Models: Predictive modeling, fueled by machine learning algorithms and sophisticated statistical analyses, is contributing to the development of precise risk prediction models for prostate cancer. These models consider a multitude of factors, including genetic markers, lifestyle variables, and environmental exposures, to generate individualized risk assessments. Such tools empower clinicians and patients with valuable information for informed decision-making and personalized preventive strategies.

8. Hormonal Therapies and Resistance Mechanisms:
Research into hormonal therapies for advanced prostate cancer is evolving, with a focus on understanding resistance mechanisms. Unraveling the molecular underpinnings of resistance allows for the development of more effective and durable hormonal treatments. Targeting specific pathways involved in resistance mechanisms holds promise for extending the effectiveness of hormonal therapies in managing advanced prostate cancer.

9. Patient-Reported Outcomes and Quality of Life:
Beyond disease-focused research, there is a growing emphasis on patient-reported outcomes and quality of life assessments. Understanding the impact of prostate health

interventions on patients' daily lives, psychological well-being, and overall satisfaction is gaining prominence. This patient-centered approach contributes to more holistic care strategies that prioritize not only disease management but also the preservation of quality of life.

In conclusion, the landscape of prostate health research is marked by an unprecedented convergence of technological innovations, molecular insights, and patient-centered paradigms. These advances hold the promise of transforming our approach to prostate health, ushering in an era of personalized medicine, targeted therapies, and improved outcomes for individuals facing prostate-related conditions. As researchers continue to unravel the complexities of prostate health, the potential for innovative breakthroughs and enhanced patient care remains on the horizon.

Promising Developments in Treatment and Prevention

In the realm of prostate health, a convergence of transformative developments has taken center stage, ushering in a new era of understanding, treatment, and prevention. As a practicing urologist, navigating this landscape involves a continuous commitment to staying informed about the latest advancements that directly impact patient care. One of the most significant strides has been witnessed in precision medicine, a paradigm shift that tailors treatments based on the unique characteristics of each individual. This approach, fueled by genomic research, has unraveled the intricate molecular tapestry of prostate conditions, particularly in the context of cancer.

Precision medicine in prostate health is not merely a theoretical concept; it is translating into tangible benefits for patients. The identification of specific genetic alterations and molecular signatures has paved the way for targeted therapies that address the underlying drivers of disease. For a urologist, this means moving beyond traditional one-size-fits-all approaches and embracing treatment plans that are personalized to the genetic makeup of each patient. The implications extend to minimizing unnecessary interventions, optimizing therapeutic outcomes, and navigating the complexities of treatment resistance with greater precision.

Immunotherapy, another beacon of hope in the landscape of prostate health, is reshaping how we approach advanced prostate cancer. As a urologist, the exploration of immune checkpoint inhibitors and therapeutic cancer vaccines has become integral to the conversation surrounding treatment modalities. Immunotherapy harnesses the body's own immune system to target and eliminate cancer cells selectively. This marks a departure from conventional treatments and holds the promise of more durable responses, offering newfound optimism for patients facing advanced stages of prostate cancer.

In the surgical arena, minimally invasive techniques continue to redefine the landscape. As a urologist, the adoption of robotic-assisted surgeries, including robot-assisted laparoscopic prostatectomy, has become standard practice. These techniques, characterized by enhanced precision and reduced recovery times, are transforming the surgical management of prostate conditions. The integration of such approaches not only aligns with the imperative for optimal patient outcomes but also reflects a commitment to embracing evolving technologies in the surgical realm.

Advanced imaging modalities have emerged as indispensable tools in the urologist's arsenal. Multiparametric magnetic resonance imaging (mpMRI) has revolutionized the diagnostic landscape, offering detailed imaging of the prostate and aiding in the targeted detection of lesions. Positron emission tomography (PET) imaging, particularly with prostate-specific membrane antigen (PSMA) tracers, is elevating the accuracy of staging and detecting recurrent disease. For a urologist, these imaging advancements translate into more precise diagnostic capabilities, informed decision-making, and improved patient outcomes.

Understanding and addressing resistance mechanisms in hormonal therapies is a key facet of contemporary urological research. For a urologist, the evolving landscape of hormonal therapies demands a nuanced approach to managing advanced prostate cancer. Research endeavors are focused on unraveling the molecular intricacies that underlie resistance, paving the way for more effective hormonal treatments. Staying abreast of these developments is essential for informed decision-making in the selection and sequencing of hormonal therapies tailored to the unique profiles of individual patients.

Radiotherapy innovations, particularly stereotactic body radiation therapy (SBRT), are reshaping the treatment paradigm for localized prostate cancer. As a urologist, incorporating these advancements into the therapeutic repertoire aligns with the imperative for precision and efficacy in radiation therapy. SBRT, characterized by its ability to deliver high doses of radiation with pinpoint accuracy, not only ensures effective disease control but also enhances patient convenience with a shorter treatment course.

Genomic testing has become a cornerstone in risk stratification for prostate cancer. As a urologist, integrating tests such as the Oncotype DX Genomic Prostate Score into the decision-making process allows for a nuanced understanding of disease aggressiveness. These tests, examining the expression of specific genes, contribute to more personalized risk assessments and inform treatment plans tailored to individual patients. Genomic testing is not merely a diagnostic tool; it has become a guiding compass in navigating the complexities of treatment decision-making.

Chemotherapy options for advanced prostate cancer have seen notable expansions, and the urologist's role in understanding and implementing these treatments is pivotal. Docetaxel and cabazitaxel have demonstrated efficacy, and ongoing research is exploring novel chemotherapeutic agents. The emphasis is not only on the development of new agents but also on identifying patient subgroups that may derive maximum benefit from specific chemotherapy regimens. For a urologist, these advancements signify a nuanced and tailored approach to chemotherapy, optimizing outcomes and quality of life for patients.

Lifestyle interventions and preventive strategies are assuming greater prominence in the urologist's toolkit. As researchers delve into the interplay between lifestyle factors, environmental exposures, and prostate health, urologists are becoming advocates for proactive preventive measures. Collaborating with patients to implement healthy lifestyle changes, such as adopting a prostate-friendly diet and engaging in regular exercise, is a proactive approach to mitigating risk factors and promoting overall well-being.

The integration of telemedicine has become a pivotal aspect of the urologist's practice, especially in the context of ongoing patient care and follow-up. As a urologist, embracing telemedicine facilitates remote consultations, follow-up appointments, and ongoing patient support. This not only enhances accessibility to healthcare services but also ensures continuity of care, particularly for patients with prostate conditions requiring monitoring and support.

In conclusion, the landscape of prostate health is undergoing a profound transformation, and the role of the urologist is evolving in tandem with these advancements. Precision medicine, immunotherapy, minimally invasive techniques, advanced imaging modalities, and a personalized approach to treatment and prevention are defining the contours of contemporary urological practice. Staying at the forefront of these developments is not merely a professional obligation for a urologist but a commitment to offering patients the highest standard of care in their journey toward prostate health and well-being.

Conclusion

Recap and Key Takeaways

In this comprehensive exploration of prostate health, the key takeaways form a cohesive narrative emphasizing a holistic and individualized approach to well-being. Lifestyle choices, from adopting a prostate-friendly diet to regular exercise, emerge as foundational in preventing prostate conditions. The paradigm-shifting concept of precision medicine is highlighted, showcasing how tailoring treatments based on individual genetic makeup optimizes therapeutic outcomes. Immunotherapy's promise in treating advanced prostate cancer represents a groundbreaking frontier, offering a potentially more effective and targeted approach. Innovations in surgical techniques, advanced imaging modalities, and evolutions in radiotherapy underscore the importance of staying at the forefront of technology in urological practice. Understanding resistance mechanisms in hormonal therapies and tailoring chemotherapy options contribute to a nuanced approach in managing advanced prostate conditions. The integration of genomic testing guides risk stratification, while lifestyle interventions play a crucial role in prevention. Telemedicine's inclusion reflects the importance of accessibility and ongoing support. In essence, this book encourages a proactive and collaborative approach, empowering both healthcare professionals and individuals to navigate the dynamic landscape of prostate health with the latest advancements and informed decision-making. Furthermore, the book underscores the transformative impact of minimally invasive surgical techniques, particularly robotic-assisted procedures, which have become standard in urological practice. These techniques not only enhance precision but also contribute to shorter recovery times, minimizing the impact on patients' lives. Advanced imaging modalities, such as multiparametric MRI and PET imaging with PSMA tracers, represent a leap forward in diagnostic capabilities, enabling urologists to make informed decisions about treatment plans and monitor prostate conditions with greater accuracy.

The nuanced understanding of resistance mechanisms in hormonal therapies, as explored in the book, is pivotal for urologists in tailoring treatments to individual patient needs. Chemotherapy developments, especially the exploration of novel agents and the identification of patient subgroups for optimized efficacy, reflect the commitment to refining therapeutic approaches and improving overall quality of life for patients with advanced prostate cancer.

Genomic testing, exemplified by the Oncotype DX Genomic Prostate Score, is presented as a guiding tool for risk stratification and personalized treatment plans. The book advocates for a proactive stance on lifestyle interventions, emphasizing not only the importance of adopting healthy habits but also quitting smoking and making dietary modifications to mitigate risk factors.

Telemedicine integration emerges as a crucial aspect, especially in providing ongoing support and follow-up for patients with prostate conditions. This reflects a commitment to accessibility and continuity of care, aligning with the evolving landscape of healthcare delivery.

In essence, the book conveys a message of empowerment and collaboration. It encourages healthcare professionals, particularly urologists, to embrace innovation, stay informed about the latest advancements, and foster a patient-centered approach that prioritizes both physical and mental well-being. By navigating the dynamic landscape of prostate health with the knowledge presented in this book, practitioners and individuals alike are equipped to make informed decisions that optimize outcomes and enhance the overall journey towards prostate health and longevity.

Looking Ahead to a Healthy Future

Looking ahead to a healthy future, the book's insights provide a roadmap for individuals, healthcare professionals, and researchers to shape a proactive and informed approach to prostate health. Emphasizing the pivotal role of preventive strategies, the importance of maintaining a prostate-friendly lifestyle through diet, exercise, and other healthy habits is underscored. The concept of precision medicine, as explored in the book, suggests a future where treatments are not only effective but specifically tailored to the genetic makeup of each individual, promising better outcomes with minimized side effects.

Immunotherapy emerges as a beacon of hope in the ongoing battle against advanced prostate cancer, pointing towards a future where the body's own immune system is harnessed for targeted and durable responses. The integration of advanced surgical techniques, such as robotic-assisted procedures, signifies a trajectory where surgeries become increasingly precise, with shorter recovery times and improved patient satisfaction.

Advanced imaging modalities, particularly multiparametric MRI and PET imaging with PSMA tracers, signal a future where diagnostic capabilities are enhanced, providing urologists with detailed insights for more accurate decision-making and monitoring of prostate conditions. Understanding and overcoming resistance mechanisms in hormonal therapies, a focal point of ongoing research, suggests a future where treatments are more tailored, addressing the specific challenges posed by advanced prostate cancer.

The book's exploration of chemotherapy developments, lifestyle interventions, genomic testing, and telemedicine integration collectively points towards a future characterized by a comprehensive and holistic approach to prostate health. By leveraging these advancements, healthcare professionals can offer more personalized care, optimizing outcomes and improving the overall quality of life for individuals navigating prostate-related conditions.

In summary, looking ahead to a healthy future in prostate health involves embracing ongoing advancements in research, technology, and patient-centered care. The book's insights serve as a foundation for envisioning a future where proactive measures, precision treatments, and innovative approaches converge to promote not only the physical but also the mental well-being of individuals. As the field continues to evolve, the collaborative efforts of researchers, healthcare professionals, and individuals alike hold the promise of shaping a future where prostate health is synonymous with longevity and overall vitality.

Appendix

Additional Resources, Websites, and Support Groups

1. Prostate Cancer Foundation (PCF): Website: Prostate Cancer Foundation The PCF is a leading organization dedicated to advancing prostate cancer research and providing comprehensive resources for patients. Their website offers a wealth of information, from the latest research updates to educational materials and support services.

2. American Urological Association (AUA): Website: American Urological Association The AUA is a reputable organization providing valuable resources for both healthcare professionals and patients. Their website features educational materials, guidelines, and information on urological conditions, including those related to the prostate.

3. Us TOO International Prostate Cancer Education and Support Network: Website: Us TOO International Us TOO is a nonprofit organization dedicated to providing support and education for men with prostate cancer and their families. The website offers resources such as support group directories, educational materials, and information on treatment options.

4. Prostate Cancer Research Institute (PCRI): Website: Prostate Cancer Research Institute The PCRI focuses on providing information about prostate cancer treatment options, ongoing research, and patient support. Their website includes video lectures, publications, and resources for individuals seeking in-depth knowledge about prostate cancer.

5. Malecare Cancer Support: Website: Malecare Cancer Support Malecare is a nonprofit organization offering support and resources for men with cancer, including prostate cancer. Their website features information on support groups, survivorship programs, and advocacy initiatives.

Support Groups:

- **Inspire Prostate Cancer Support Community:** Website: Inspire Prostate Cancer Community Inspire is an online platform hosting a prostate cancer support community where individuals can connect, share experiences, and seek advice from others navigating similar journeys.

- **Reddit - Prostate Cancer Community:** Subreddit: r/ProstateCancer Reddit's Prostate Cancer community provides a forum for individuals to ask questions, share stories, and receive support from a diverse group of individuals who have experienced or are currently facing prostate cancer.

- **CancerCare Prostate Cancer Online Support Group:** Website: CancerCare Prostate Cancer Support Group CancerCare offers online support groups for prostate cancer patients and their loved ones. These groups provide a safe space for sharing experiences and gaining insights into coping with the challenges of prostate cancer.

These resources, websites, and support groups collectively contribute to a robust network of information, education, and emotional support for individuals navigating prostate health challenges. They represent a forward-looking approach to promoting a healthy future by ensuring that individuals have access to comprehensive and reliable resources as they manage their prostate health journey.